HEALTH WITH A MISSION

Lose Weight by Gaining Health: Twelve
Weeks of Personal Transformation

WILLIAM B. HAYNES

WESTBOW
PRESS

WestBow Press books may be ordered through booksellers or by contacting:

WestBow Press
A Division of Thomas Nelson
1663 Liberty Drive
Bloomington, IN 47403
www.westbowpress.com
1-(866) 928-1240

Because of the dynamic nature of the Internet, any Web addresses or links contained in this book may have changed since publication and may no longer be valid. The views expressed in this work are solely those of the author and do not necessarily reflect the views of the publisher, and the publisher hereby disclaims any responsibility for them.

ISBN: 978-1-4497-0201-4 (sc)
ISBN: 978-1-4497-0203-8 (hc)
ISBN: 978-1-4497-0202-1 (e)

Library of Congress Control Number: 2010927359

For further information, please contact:

William Haynes
NuLifeRx, LLC
550 Brookwood Point Place
Simpsonville, SC 29681
(864) 688-1045

William@nuliferx.com

Scripture quoted by permission. Quotations designated (NET) are from the NET Bible® copyright ©1996-2006 by Biblical Studies Press, L.L.C. www.bible.org All rights reserved.

Printed in the United States of America
WestBow Press rev. date: 8/10/2010

Contents

Acknowledgements

I'd like to thank my incredible wife and partner, Cindy Haynes, for her love, dedication, and support during the many hours of writing this book. As we were both going through our weight loss transformation, her insights gave the ideas for several lessons this book.

I want to thank my savior Jesus Christ, through whom all things are possible. His saving grace and redemptive love brought me through the tough times and helped me regain balance and health in my life.

Simpsonville First Baptist Church has been incredibly supportive throughout our time on the mission field and in supporting this fitness project. Our family has been blessed to be a part of this great church body.

My friends at NuLifeRx have been an incredible encouragement to me. This is an amazing group of health and fitness professionals who understand "Health With A Mission" and are helping spread the word! A special thanks to Mike Worley who helped finding the perfect scriptures for each chapter.

I am thankful that God is One who gives second chances and an opportunity for redemption. The joy of being in a healthy body is boundless.

My thanks to the Biblical Studies Press who granted permission for their NET Bible to be quoted in this book. This Bible is available in its entirety as a free download or online at http://www.nextbible.org.

Many thanks also to the Will Graham and my friends at the Billy Graham Evangelistic Association for allowing me to print their "Steps to Peace with God" in the Appendix of this book.

A Letter from Steve Newman, MD

"I urge you, brothers, in view of God's mercy, to offer your bodies as living sacrifices, holy and pleasing to God – this is your spiritual act of worship." Romans 12:1

God's word often references the value of health and wellness. There is a basic responsibility that each of us must accept when it comes to our individual well being. Sadly, the fundamental principles of routine exercise and proper nutrition are too often ignored and willfully neglected. Obesity is epidemic in our country, afflicting over 2/3 of our adult population. Equally disturbing is the fact that the segment of our population demonstrating the fastest growing percentage of obesity is children. Excessive weight unequivocally contributes to many of our nation's leading causes of death; including diabetes, heart disease, stroke and a myriad of cancers. Imagine the incredible influence which could occur if individuals gained a greater sense of self accountability and focused their attention on improving nutrition, participating in regular exercise and maintaining an appropriate weight. Such success begins with a simple, yet sincere, desire for change.

"For I know the plans I have for you says the Lord. They are plans for good and not for evil, to give you a future and a hope." Jeremiah 29:11

The journey of gaining health is one which requires a lifetime of commitment and discipline. For too truly gain health one must make changes involving both personal habits and lifestyle – choices which are to be woven into the very fabric of one's being. This is precisely the reason many diets and weight loss programs fail as they do not address the need to structure dynamic change within a person's life, habits and knowledge base.

The book you are about to begin should be used as a tool, a road map if you will, toward obtaining such knowledge. Use it to propel yourself forward targeting the ultimate goal of gaining health and improving your life. To do so will be one of the most important acts you will ever undertake. Good health is a blessing and a gift from God - one which we should do all within our power to nurture and maintain. May God bless you in your efforts and to Him, always, be the glory.

"Dr. Nu"
Dr. Steve Newman
NuLifeRx – Greenville, SC

Health With A Mission

You're not on this earth by accident. You are here for a purpose and designed with a mission for life. Whether your mission is in the overseas mission field, raising your family as a great mom, Sunday school teacher or football coach, you need a healthy body to accomplish your mission to its full extent.

Does your body reflect God's marvelous design? I hope so! He designed your body with amazing muscles and possibilities for movement! How have you done as a caretaker? Like the servant with the talents in Matthew 25:14-30, God gave each of us assets to tend. Some take these assets and multiply them, creating even more than they had been given. Some bury it in the ground and do nothing with it.

Your God gave you a body, an asset to care for. What have you done with that asset?

- Developed your body into an athletic form, able to do more today than you were years ago.
- Maintained your body so that you're not much better off, or worse, than you were years ago.
- Taken poor care of your body so that it's worse off than years ago.

If the answer is anything but the first choice, then it's time to change. Start living *Health With A Mission* and develop this gift of life that God's given you. Through physical health, we have the ability to accomplish our mission on earth, whatever God has called us to.

As I discovered, it's not too late for redemption! Whether you've been "maintaining" or your body is severely out of shape, God has designed your body to respond quickly to healthy change. By the end of this twelve week program, you'll see muscles and abilities that you may have only dreamed of on day one!

What is Sabai Fitness?

Sabai is a Thai word which means peaceful and healthy. When I set out to start my fitness company, I looked for a name that expressed my vision. Sabai Fitness will challenge you to create these: Peace with the Creator; Peace with your mission; and Health in your body. At Sabai Fitness, we promote and encourage great health based on God's design for life.

Your journey to health will be a process of gaining a healthy mind and body. Gaining weight was as much a mental process as a physical process... so is gaining health.

Whether or not you are at your optimum physical shape, you can have Sabai Fitness by developing health. Sabai Fitness isn't about a diet or a specific exercise program. It's about using natural and common-sense strategies to gain health and peace within our lives. By focusing on the natural and simple process of becoming healthy; we create habits which support our body for a vibrant and happy life. We can then use our vibrant life to bless and serve others.

Sabai Fitness partners with a wonderful company called NuLifeRx, which is a group of medical professionals with a similar vision. We work with individuals wanting one-on-one coaching and with groups doing the "Health With A Mission" plan. You can check NuLifeRx out at www.nuliferx.com.

Let us know if we can work with you or your company to develop a custom and effective fitness program that supports health and vitality. Contact the author at william@sabaifitness.com . You can explore Sabai Fitness and find more information at www.sabaifitness.com.

How this works

This book is your coach in the process of gaining health. You won't find a series of specific exercises and diets. Why? Part of the process is finding what works well for you body. You will find common sense and truth that will help you find your way and develop a lifestyle of health. I'm honored that you chose this book to help you in the journey.

This book is a series of lessons over 12 weeks designed to be read daily and applied to your life. While you could read through them all or skip around, the book has been written for you to work through one lesson and journal each day. By completing the lessons and applying the concepts to your life, you'll find that you have gained tremendous health during these 12 weeks!

The lessons are cumulative and the start may seem slow, but quickly you will be applying the lessons together and making huge changes in your life and mindset. The goal of this book is to help you make the real changes that need to happen for you to gain health and maintain it long-term. I promise that you will receive from this book in direct proportion that you work the plan.

Prayer partners and friends who are committed to this same process will be an incredible support system. If you don't have anyone going through this program with you, come to www.healthwithamission.com and connect with some new friends on this journey. Learn to lean on them, sharing your successes and challenges. We are the Body of Christ and interdependent on each other.

Your current physical condition is a reflection of your beliefs and actions. The book addresses both of these areas. By addressing beliefs and actions that need to be changes to gain health, we create tangible steps to create change.

Let this book be your coach and trust the process. Do one lesson each day and focus on that day. The lesson is done when you complete the journal. If you miss a day, don't stress, just pick up with the missed lesson and move on. Stumbling doesn't mean failure, just a short delay. Gaining health is not a race with a finish line, but a process which is life-long. It will find its own "healthy" weight, as you make these changes. I pray you gain fitness as you take your journey. May you develop a sense of peace, serenity, and health during your journey and come closer to Christ.

Components of this Process

Health With A Mission – The Book

Lessons –Twelve weeks of daily principles to apply

Journal – Daily journal entries where you apply the lesson to your life.

Support:

Online Community – We've set up an online community to encourage and support each other. Use this as a place to connect during the week, blog about what you've learned, and cheer each other on. To join, go online to www.healthwithamission.com

Small Group – Consider creating a small group where you can share this journey together. A small group is a safe place for you to connect with others, share successes and encourage each other through challenges. Contact us for support materials at www.healthwithamission.com.

Prayer partner – Talk with a friend and ask them to be your prayer partner. A prayer partner praying for you each day during the 12 weeks, lifting up your concerns and giving praise for your successes will help you tremendously. Let your prayer partner know how to best pray for you. Consider getting them a book as well, so they can be praying specifically for you.

Church – This can be a powerful study for a church body to go through together. If your church is considering this study for a large group or congregation, please contact me. I'll help in any way I can to help you make it a success.

Discounts are available for bulk purchases over 20 books:

Contact: William Haynes – william@sabaifitness.com

William's Story

It seems that I was always a "big guy," but in retrospect I realize that isn't really true. I became a big guy sometime during my freshman year in college. Before that, I was more the thin, geeky type that always looked a little uncomfortable in my own skin.

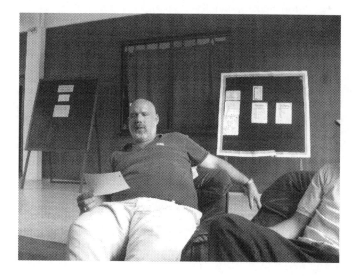

Over the years, the pounds piled on. I was 212 pounds as a freshman in college and later moved into the higher two hundreds. I remained there for much of my adult life. In 2004, I put 285 lbs on my driver's license because the Department of Motor Vehicles didn't check. Even though I already weighed more than 300 pounds, I figured it was close enough!

In 1999, after a business failure, the scales began to move up again. Eating anything that looked good combined with a sedentary lifestyle resulted in a waistline that was ever expanding. I had moved from a 32-inch waist as a teen to seeking 54 inch waist pants in discount stores as an adult. Why would you want to pay full price for something that looked so bad?

In September of 2007, I was tired and fed up. I weighed 359 lbs. I was "morbidly obese". I was sick of being fat. That day, I committed to a strict diet and dropped nine pounds by the end of the month. Rather than being excited by my weight loss, I was frustrated and angry. Dieting was a painful process and the long road ahead looked bleak.

I turned to God in prayer. "Dear Lord… I can't do this on my own! Please help me!" God gently whispered, "Gain Health. Quit worrying about losing weight." This shift has made a world of difference and paved the way toward success and happiness.

By focusing on health, I started making better decisions and learning lessons that created fitness. In the process, the pounds started coming off! Nine months after beginning my quest for health, I ran a Sprint distance triathlon (750 m swim, 20 km bike, and 5 km run). Over 100 pounds came off while doing regular exercise and eating well.

I haven't "dieted" since my shift to gaining health, though; I have drastically changed the way I eat! The focus is on eating healthy foods and snacks that build my energy. The further I've come in this journey, the more I realize that "diets" can be counter-productive to gaining health. I realize that changing my eating and exercise was only a part of the journey that I needed to take. To make long term changes, I needed to address the beliefs and actions that created my obese condition.

It's hard to describe how much better my life is today. I feel lighter on my feet and I am, quite literally. I am balanced and poised when I walk. I am amazed at the little things, like being able to pick something up off the floor, just by leaning over.

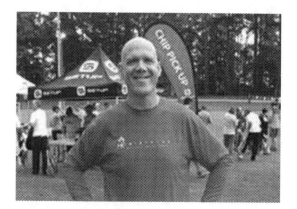

Running is something I love and I am a triathlete. I've cycled 60 miles in four hours and gone windsurfing during vacation. Two years after I began this journey, I completed the Ironman Augusta 70.3 triathlon. Life is no longer something I'm trudging through, but an experience I'm embracing. Whether things are going well or are challenging, I see both as opportunities to develop different aspects of my character. The thing that has most surprised me is how the physical carries over to other areas in life. Since gaining health, I've gained a bright and optimistic mental outlook, and I've developed spiritual depth as well. My lifelong goal of writing a book has been achieved and I'm fulfilling my drive to help others.

Embrace this opportunity! Make today the turning point from which everything changes. I'll hold your hand through the process and help you succeed. Choose health!

PART I: SABAI CORE –
BASICS MAKE THE DIFFERENCE

My child, pay attention to my words; listen attentively to my sayings. Do not let them depart from your sight, guard them within your heart; for they are life to those who find them and healing to one's entire body. Proverbs 4:20-22 (NET)

No matter how frustrated you may be with your current state of health, today is the day that things begin to change.

Sabai is a Thai word for health, wellness, peace, and contentment. We really cannot have these without Christ. He is the center of all that is good. My prayer for you is to experience a deepening of your relationship with Christ as you embrace the healthy principles that God designed for your life.

The Sabai CORE is a set of the basics that you need for great health. If these four components are present in your life, you'll find the weight coming off. This process of consistent focus on the basics will help you gain health and in the process create the weight loss you've dreamed of. Embrace this opportunity! Take advantage of this day to turn toward the design that God created in your body... a design of beauty, strength, and health.

Let's focus on God's original design and seek His wisdom. Through this focus we begin healing our body. We don't need to create something new but discover what has always existed.

You will get out of this process a result proportional to your input. A poor effort will give a poor result. An excellent effort will yield an excellent result! The choice is yours and today is decision time. Decide to commit the next 12 weeks. Decide to complete each day's tasks. Commit to completing each journal entry.

Remember, the lesson is complete when the journal is completed. Shortcuts will not create the change you're seeking. By doing each lesson fully and applying it to your life through the journaling process, you'll see tremendous change. By committing to the process, you're setting yourself up for success!

WEEK 1 DAY 1: *Know Where You Stand*

Make the path for your feet level, so that all your ways may be established. Proverbs 4:26 (NET)

As you begin a journey, it's crucial to understand where you're starting from. It is important to take a snapshot of your starting fitness level which will give you foundation for the changes ahead.

This journey will be based on finding the truth about yourself, your body, and how you were created to be. If you avoid the truth of your present condition, you also avoid progress. By having a clear picture of your current weight, clothing size, and physical ability, you can mark the starting line and see the changes as your body gains health.

Want to know how to succeed? Success is created through consistent movement toward a goal.

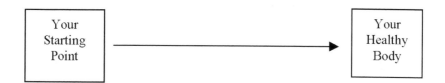

If you are in one city and your goal is in another city, you can get there many ways. A taxi may get you there faster than walking, but either way, consistent movement toward the goal is virtually guaranteed to get you there.

Take steps each day to gain health and move away from an unhealthy lifestyle. You will get there! Focus on the successes you have created. These can include drinking enough water, exercising, doing other physical activities, proper rest, or eating a healthy meal. Each one of these gets you closer to your goal and should be acknowledged as a success.

Spend your energy and focus on the process rather than the end destination. You'll get there soon enough. Don't miss the wonderful journey along the way. Your goal is consistent movement towards the goal. Acknowledge your progress when you have had a tough day. By acknowledging your progress, you are doing a reality check that will encourage continued change.

Get a clear picture of your starting point and commit to constant daily movement toward your fitness goals!

Week 1 Day 1: *Initial Measurements*

Today's Date:___/___/___

Weight:_____

Get an accurate weight by using a quality scale. If you weigh more than your present scale can handle, then your local hospital or health care provider should be able to help you get your initial weight.

Map out a one mile distance. Walk, jog, or run this distance at your best pace. Record the time.

One mile speed:_____

Waist:_____

Record your waist size using a measuring tape or record your pant size.

Chest:_____

Record your chest size using a measuring tape or record your shirt size.

Remember, this is your starting point. It's important to know where you are before you start heading toward your destination!

Take a photograph to record your current look.

 Check the box when you've done this.

Place Your Photo Here

Write down other measurements you'd like to record: (example: bust, thigh, arm, bench press, anything you want!)

Congratulations, when you've finished these measurements and written them down, you've finished Day One!

WEEK 1 DAY 2: *Gain Health!*

Finally, brothers and sisters, whatever is true, whatever is worthy of respect, whatever is just, whatever is pure, whatever is lovely, whatever is commendable, if something is excellent or praiseworthy, think about these things. Philippians 4:8 (NET)

Consider this verse from Philippians and how it applies to your journey of gaining health. Committing to health makes a lot more sense that committing to weight loss. Health is excellent and praiseworthy!

Symptoms are sometimes confused with the problem. The weight is the symptom while the problem is being unhealthy. Let's focus on a solution that addresses the problem and builds health into your life. A healthy body naturally maintains a great weight and supports an active life. This is the basis of the Sabai CORE. Over the next several days, you will learn the Sabai CORE that will help you create this health in your life.

When we focus on health, our choices change. Health is about eating fresh veggies and fruits, quality proteins and whole grains, exercising regularly, spending time outside, and spending time with family and friends in great activities. Health means bringing our body back into God's original design. God created us all with strength, resilience, and possibility. A life based on God's design is a life filled with opportunity and excitement.

By pursuing God's best for our life and body, we naturally change parts of our life that do not fit into that design. What are some things that do not fit into God's original design?

- Excess body weight
- Unhealthy foods
- Lack of movement
- Embracing an identity as damaged or less than others

Let's start focusing on gaining health! Gaining health reflect God's design is our goal and focus. Start making choices that support health and vibrancy in your life! In the process of gaining health, your body's weight will come back into balance and your life will begin reflecting God's design. Gain health!

WEEK 1 DAY 2: *Journal*

List some choices that you've been making that have damaged your health. Commit to stopping or limiting these choices. Examples include: Smoking; cookies during your morning coffee break; three hours of television at night.

_____

_____

_____

These actions have been moving you away from your goal. They've destroyed health rather than built into it. Choose new actions which will take you toward your goal.

What are three actions that you will take consistently to move you closer to your goal? For example: Get to bed before 10 pm each night or eating fresh veggies or fruit with every meal.

_____

_____

_____

By focusing on consistent progress, you move away from the "all or nothing" mentality that can set up a cycle of failure. Rather than "all or nothing", its "slow and steady" that wins the race.

People who are successful make consistent progress toward their outcomes. A key to achieving long-term weight loss is having attained it through consistent and persistent action.

Occasionally, we have those "breakthrough" days where huge progress is gained. Many days there is minor progress toward the goal and those small steps is what success is made of! That's what we're striving for!

WEEK 1 DAY 3: *Your Pivot Point*

That we, being rescued from the hand of our enemies, may serve him without fear, in holiness and righteousness before him for as long as we live. Luke 1:74-75 (NET)

In each person's life, there are pivot points. The most important of these pivot points is the day that we choose to follow Christ and become His disciple. We turn away from living for self and turn toward relationship with our Savior.

These pivot points are critical. As long as we're heading in the wrong direction we are guaranteed bad results. As soon as we turn and commit to God's plan for our life, we can begin working toward success.

I had a pivot point on September 30th, 2007. I realized the problem wasn't my weight but my lack of health. I was extremely unhealthy and the weight was a symptom of the problem, not the problem itself. On that date, I started working toward making healthy choices in my life and my life was changed. My problems weren't gone, but I had begun making consistent progress toward their solution!

Looking back in my notes, I started very simply by walking 20 minutes a day. My unhealthy condition wasn't created in a day, and the solution wouldn't be created immediately either.

I have read that the average person makes hundreds of food choices in a day. I believe it! Those of us who have gained weight through the years have made too many unhealthy choices. The balance needs to shift to making healthy choices rather than unhealthy ones.

Have you had a "pivot point"? By choosing this book and deciding to commit to the 12 weeks, you can make this your pivot point. Working these lessons into your life is a natural pivot point when you choose to make it one.

This means that you've got to make the decision to change. Say it out loud if you've decided to gain health! Remind yourself throughout the day that life has changed and you are gaining health!

Create your pivot point today!

WEEK 1 DAY 3: *Journal*

Today's verse reminds us that it is God who rescues us, so that we may serve him without fear. The day that we lean into God and begin to rely on His help creates a pivot point. As mentioned before, the first month I spent dieting on my own will power. It was only after I cried out to God for him that he rescued me.

What are some pivot points that you've had in your life? These are moments in time after which things changed forever. For example: The day I met my spouse, the day I began college, the moment I chose to quit smoking.

_____

_____

_____

Each pivot point helps create a new outcome down the road. Notice the results that happened because of the pivot points you've already had in your life.

Working through this book daily and working through the journals will create a new pivot point in your life. After working through this book, things will be changed forever! List three outcomes that you expect after a year of continuing down this new path. For example: Clothes fit me well; I feel strong; I sleep well at night.

_____

_____

_____

Put a star by the outcome that you're most excited about having in your life!

WEEK 1 DAY 4: *The Sabai CORE*

For this is the way God loved the world: He gave his one and only Son, so that everyone who believes in him will not perish but have eternal life. For God did not send his Son into the world to condemn the world, but that the world should be saved through him. John 3:16-17 (NET)

Your body needs four cornerstones for a solid health foundation. This is what I call the Sabai CORE:

C – Cardio Movement

O - Optimum Hydration

R - Rest and Recovery

E - Eat Healthy

Cardio Movement – Cardio exercise that strengthens your heart is the foundation of your body's fitness. The movement gained by cardio is critical for a healthy body. Our body was made for movement, and we increase our health by exercising daily and adding motion to our day. With movement, the body's lymph system flushes toxins from our body and helps us fight disease.

Optimum Hydration – The human body consists of up to 75% water. Your body needs optimum hydration to function properly. When you exercise regularly and particularly when you are losing weight, the need for water is increased. The breakdown of fat creates byproducts that need to be flushed from the body. Drinking water throughout the day is the best way to achieve optimum hydration!

Rest and Recovery – By exercising regularly, your body has demands placed on it during the day. Your time of sleep helps you recover from those demands. Many people don't put any physical demands on their body during the day and then wonder why they can't sleep at night! By incorporating cardio movement into your day, you'll welcome sleep and develop a great pattern of rest and recovery.

Eat Healthy – The quality of the foods that you are putting in your body is crucial to gaining health. Eating vegetables and fruit, whole grains, lean proteins, and less processed foods builds your energy and health. By eating natural foods, your energy level will increase and you will cleanse what is unwanted from your body.

Remember, Sabai means health, wellness, peace, and contentment. By developing your Sabai CORE, you'll develop health in your life.

WEEK 1 DAY 4: *Journal*

The Sabai CORE is the foundation for a healthy body. How would you currently rate your body in these areas?

Rate these on a scale of 1 to 10 with 1 being the worst and 10 being excellent

C – Cardio Movement_____

O - Optimum Hydration_____

R - Rest and Recovery_____

E – Eat Healthy _____

Whichever got the lowest score should be a special area of focus. The reason is that this area is the easiest to make significant change in! When I am training for my triathlons, the weakest area is the one where I spend the most time and study. I love making significant progress and this speeds the process.

Journal your Sabai CORE each day. You can continue to grade on a scale of 1 to 10. Also, jot down what you did and how did it work? This process of tracking the Sabai CORE will give you benchmarks and help you learn from your efforts.

✦ Today's Sabai CORE:

C – Cardio Movement _____

O – Optimum Hydration _____

R – Rest and Recovery _____

E – Eat Healthy _____

WEEK 1 DAY 5: *C - Cardio Movement*

I run along the path of your commands, for you enable me to do so. Psalm 119:32 (NET)

Your body was designed to move. Cardio exercise requires constant movement over time. Cardio exercise strengthens your heart and helps increase its output in every beat. Walking is a great cardio exercise, as is running, biking, and swimming. You can also do cardio in the gym by doing time on the treadmill, the elliptical machine, the rower, or the Stairmaster. The heart will strengthen and your muscles will become stronger.

A body needs to be challenged, or it becomes weakened. Many people act as if their body is like a car with a limited amount of mileage. They keep it garaged as much as possible by spending their day sitting and lethargic. Instead of a mechanical system, like a car, your body is an organic system. Things in nature are in a process of growing and strengthening or weakening and dying. Let's stay growing and strengthening!

Lifting weights is also a wonderful way to increase your strength, but without a cardio foundation, you can gain muscle without having a healthy core. Start with cardio movement and get your foundation strong. Focus first on your Sabai CORE foundation. When your body starts strengthening, then add weight work to get the definition that you are looking for!

While the goal of some people is to move as little as possible during the day, your goal is the opposite. Move as much as possible during the day! A focused cardio workout gives you movement, and so does walking during your daily activities. Your body was made for motion. The more often you can get your body up and moving, the healthier you'll be.

When you do cardio movement, you burn calories as your metabolism increases. The great thing is that your metabolism continues to run at an increased rate even after your exercise! You've lit the fire and it continues to burn long after you finish the exercise. Your increase in daily metabolism will keep excess weight dropping off your body.

Move!

Week 1 Day 5: *Journal*

Consider today's scripture and how it applies to living healthy. Jot down some thoughts about how this applies in your life.

_____

_____

Cardio movement will strengthen your heart as you exercise your body. Any motion that is continuous over time can be used as your cardio workout. These exercises include walking, running, biking, swimming, skiing, treadmill, Stairmaster, rowing, skipping rope, jumping on a trampoline, jumping jacks, hiking, raking leaves, and many others. What are your three favorite cardio exercises? You don't have to love them yet, but these are your top three.

1. _____

2. _____

3. _____

Put a star next to one of these cardio movements that you'll do today as part of your Sabai CORE. Do it as long as you have fun with it. Fifteen minutes is a great start, or you can do it longer. Focus on what you like about it and why you chose it to be in your top three. Does it get you outside? Are you able to do it with your kids, friends, or spouse? Connect with what makes it a great exercise for you!

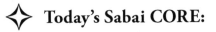 Today's Sabai CORE:

C – Cardio Movement   _____

O – Optimum Hydration   _____

R – Rest and Recovery   _____

E – Eat Healthy   _____

WEEK 1 DAY 6: *Beginning Cardio*

I know, Lord, that your regulations are just. You disciplined me because of your faithful devotion to me. Psalm 119:76 (NET)

How do you get started with cardio? Start off simply by committing to two, three, or four 15 minute blocks of cardio every day. By starting simply and in small blocks, you set yourself up for success.

In the beginning, I chose a goal of exercising an hour a day. The problem was that I couldn't exercise for an hour straight without WAY overdoing it. I was sore, tired, and ready to quit before I really got started. Something had to change and that change was using 15 minute blocks. By breaking the hour of exercise into four 15 minute blocks, I started having fun and succeeding. What a difference that made! My hour of exercise could be:

- 15 minute walk during lunch
- 15 minutes bike ride after work
- 30 minutes of active Wii games with the boys in the evening

Everyone can find the time for exercise, if they can break the time into smaller blocks. It's your body, so you make the rules! Consider the activities that you could do to make your cardio time each day:

- Go swimming with your kids
- Take a brisk walk
- Lift weights
- Go for a run
- Ride your bike
- Play a high activity Wii game
- Do Tae Bo or other exercise video

- Jump Rope
- Go hiking
- Walk at the mall

Whether you start with a half hour, forty-five minutes, or an hour, you'll be exercising consistently and wanting more!

Week 1 Day 6: *Journal*

The Lord disciplines us because of his devotion to our development. You discipline your body for the same reason. Without discipline, the human body can never reach its God given potential. With discipline, you'll see your body begin to shape and change in ways that God intended.

Fifteen-minute blocks allow you to break your exercise down into chunks that you can manage. By creating these blocks during the day and doing the exercises that you choose, your process of gaining health becomes fun and achievable. Choose from two to four fifteen-minute blocks that you'll commit to today. You can do the same activity for several of the blocks if you want. You can also do some blocks back-to-back. It's your body, your program, and you make the rules!

15 Minute Blocks

1. _____

2. _____

3. _____

4. _____

Enjoy your cardio today and have fun with your fifteen-minute blocks. Feel free to invite someone else along.

◆ Today's Sabai CORE:

C – Cardio Movement _____

O – Optimum Hydration _____

R – Rest and Recovery _____

E – Eat Healthy _____

WEEK 1 DAY 7: *Add Movement to your Routine*

But those who wait for the LORD's help find renewed strength; they rise up as if they had eagles' wings, they run without growing weary, they walk without getting tired. Isaiah 40:31 (NET)

Add movement into your daily routine. For example, when you're heading to the grocery store, where do you park? Most people drive around in circles to find the closest parking spot… Why? This is a habit that is counterproductive to our goal of health.

You benefit in several ways by parking on the other side of the parking lot. While it is further from the store, you get these benefits:

- You save the fuel cost of driving in circles.
- You don't look silly waiting like a vulture for an open spot.
- You save your car from door dings.
- You have a quicker path out when you're finished shopping.
- You get exercise by walking across the parking lot.

It just makes sense to park and walk. Find other ways to add movement to your day.

- Take the stairs
- Walk during lunch break
- Park on the far side of a parking lot
- Take short walk breaks during your workday.
- Rake the yard
- Ride your bike
- Mop the floor
- Explore downtown

This is one of the fastest ways to make fitness a regular state of mind!

WEEK 1 DAY 7: *Journal*

List ten ways to add movement to your day. Be creative and begin changing your habits. See how many you can come up with that you can incorporate into your routine. You can use any from the lesson that you can apply to your life. See if you can come up with 10!

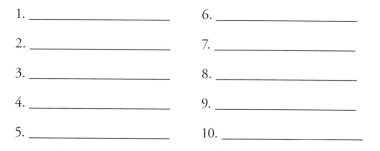

1. _____   6. _____

2. _____   7. _____

3. _____   8. _____

4. _____   9. _____

5. _____   10. _____

Pick a few of these to do today and have fun with it! Be creative with all the ways that you can add some movement to your day. By moving, you're increasing your metabolism and will find that you have more energy throughout your day.

As you find some activities that you are really excited about doing, it will be less of a chore. Today's verse promises renewed strength when we focus on the Lord.

✦ Today's Sabai CORE:

C – Cardio Movement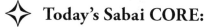

O – Optimum Hydration   _____

R – Rest and Recovery   _____

E – Eat Healthy   _____

Week 2 Day 1: *O - Optimum Hydration*

"But whoever drinks some of the water that I will give him will never be thirsty again, but the water that I will give him will become in him a fountain of water springing up to eternal life."
John 4:14 (NET)

Optimum Hydration means having the water your body needs so that your cells and organs function properly. It is vital to drink water throughout the day and even more so when you are losing weight.

Water is the most common molecule in your body, making up about two-thirds of your mass. This molecule is crucial in functions ranging from cellular energy, to oxygen transport, to cleansing toxins from your body.

When you exercise, you increase your body's demand for water in three ways. First, you are releasing water through each increased breath you're taking. Second, you are sweating and losing water through the perspiration. Third, you are building up toxins from muscle use and the fat breakdown that need to be cleansed from your body with water.

The amount of water that you need will depend somewhat on your local climate and the amount of exercise that you are doing. Being dehydrated limits your ability to exercise and will increase the time you need for recovery.

During the day drink at least six to eight .5 liter bottles of water. On a hot day, when doing outside activities, you'll need to increase your water intake. You can know if you're getting enough water by noticing the color of your urine. You should be urinating multiple times each day and the color should be a clear to light yellow. When the urine starts getting darker, then you need to drink more water.

As the weeks go by, your body will adjust to having enough water readily available. You will notice if you've forgotten to drink your water because you won't feel the same health and strength that you do when you're properly hydrated.

There are two other signs of inadequate water consumption: headaches and hunger. Water helps to keep both these at bay!

WEEK 2 DAY 1: *Journal*

Drinking water throughout the day is critical to developing health and wellness. Water bathes our cells, keeps our blood flowing well and carrying oxygen throughout our body, and helps clean toxins away from our muscles and cells through the lymph system. By maintaining optimum hydration, you're setting your body up for health! What were the top three drinks you consumed prior to today? Were they natural or processed? Example: Diet Soda – Processed, Fresh Orange Juice – Natural

Food Item   Natural or Processed?

1. _____   _____

2. _____   _____

3. _____   _____

Your best drink during the day is water and you can supplement this with natural drinks, such as juices or milk. A great rule of thumb is the fresher, the better!

Jesus talked about being the living water. It's an example of how crucial water is to our lives. In Genesis 1:1-2, after God created the heavens and earth, the spirit of God moved over the water before land and sky were made. When he wanted life in the Garden of Eden, he created springs of water.

Water was created by God to nourish life. Drink it and enjoy it with thanksgiving.

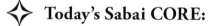 **Today's Sabai CORE:**

C – Cardio Movement   _____

O – Optimum Hydration   _____

R – Rest and Recovery   _____

E – Eat Healthy   _____

Week 2 Day 2: R - Rest and Recovery

> *By the seventh day God finished the work that he had been doing, and he ceased on the seventh day all the work that he had been doing. Genesis 2:2 (NET)*

Rest and recovery are part of the Sabai CORE for a reason! They are critical to your health. A healthy body makes demands on its muscles, organs, and systems. A time of rest gives the body time to recover and grow strong.

As you see in the title for this lesson, there are two main components to this area, rest and recovery. By rest, I'm referring to your sleep. For your body to be healthy, it needs that downtime at night to recover from the day and strengthen for the day ahead. This is also a time for your brain to process and integrate the lessons learned that day. If you don't give yourself adequate time to sleep, you're cheating yourself.

During the week, you should have a recovery day to give your body an opportunity to rest and strengthen. Working out is healthy unless your body doesn't ever get a chance to recover. There's a reason why God rested on the seventh day. It's healthy to! Give yourself permission to rest. If life is in constant overdrive, you limit your fun and increase your chances for injury.

Your recovery day is a break from focused exercise, but it's not a cheat day! I once was on a diet (unsuccessfully) that allowed for a cheat day each week. That didn't work for me at all! I'd plan all week how much unhealthy food I could pack into that one day.

Learn to relax, rest and recover. Your recovery day is just part of being healthy, not a departure from your healthy habits. Eat well, drink your water, and get your rest. If you feel like doing light activities, feel free, but give yourself a break from heavy exercise. Healthy living is something we do every day and rest is part of living healthy!

If God chose to rest on the seventh day, wouldn't it be wise for you to make the same choice?

Week 2 Day 2: *Journal*

By constantly taking note of how the journey is going and making minor adjustments where needed, you're setting a pattern for success. Feel free to write notes in the margins at any time you want to record a feeling, a new record, or just want to capture something in the moment! Jot down some thoughts about the first week of your journey. What has been easier than you expected? What is an area where you've realized that you need to improve?

Journal:

_____

_____

Acknowledge that the first steps can be the toughest. Your hardest week is the one that you've already completed. Once you've gotten started and begin developing momentum, the journey becomes a natural and exciting part of life.

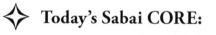 **Today's Sabai CORE:**

C – Cardio Movement   _____

O – Optimum Hydration   _____

R – Rest and Recovery   _____

E – Eat Healthy   _____

Week 2 Day 3: $\mathcal{E}$ – Eat Healthy

Daniel 1:12-13 "Please test your servants for ten days by providing us with some vegetables to eat and water to drink. Then compare our appearance with that of the young men who are eating the royal delicacies; deal with us in light of what you see." (NET)

My "food pyramid" looks a lot different than the model we grew up with... in fact, it's upside-down! Start from the top and eat your way down the pyramid, choosing 75% or more of your foods within the top few layers and only occasionally choosing foods from the bottom half of the pyramid. Let's take a look:

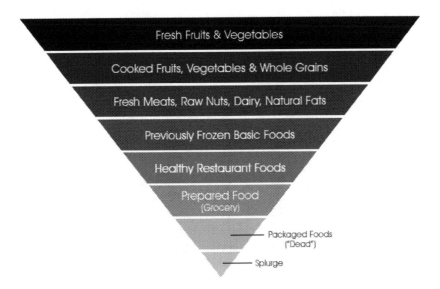

I've always loved food and even share recipes with others on cooking websites. Dieting was like torture for me. Eating healthy isn't! Eating healthy means fresh veggies and fruit, fresh meats, nuts, and dairy in my meals. What's to complain about that?

Tomorrow, I'll break down the categories, but for now just notice the pattern: lots of fresh and natural foods prepared in your own kitchen and very few packaged or prepared foods. Perhaps you are concerned that you don't have the time to cook. No worries… Come to www.sabaifitness.com and check out the recipes and menu links.

There are several diets out there that focus on fresh fruits and vegetables, whole grains, and naturally healthy foods. The challenge is that a diet tends to be an unnatural structure. If you choose to follow a weight loss diet, make sure it works with this food pyramid. The goal is to develop a lifestyle of choosing great foods that support health. You'll create a strong Sabai CORE by eating foods that are healthy. It's that simple.

Week 2 Day 3: *Journal*

In our verse today, notice how Daniel wasn't looking for a low carb diet or a special protein shake to make him healthy. He wanted the things that God had designed for his body rather than the rich food from the royal court. Within 10 days there was already enough of a difference for it to be noticeable! You can look online and see there are diets designed that are based on this scripture.

Write down everything you eat today and decide where each item goes in the food pyramid. Is it in the top half, where you want the vast majority of your food, or in the bottom half that you want to minimize? Use another sheet or write in the margins if you run out of room.

Today's Foods:

Item   Pyramid Location (Top/Bottom)

_____   _____

_____   _____

_____   _____

_____   _____

_____   _____

You want 75% or more of your foods coming from the top half of the pyramid.

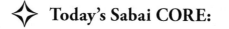 **Today's Sabai CORE:**

C – Cardio Movement _____

O – Optimum Hydration _____

R – Rest and Recovery _____

E – Eat Healthy _____

Week 2 Day 4: *Eat for Health – Top Four!*

Now without faith it is impossible to please him, for the one who approaches God must believe that he exists and that he rewards those who seek him. Hebrews 11:6 (NET)

Let's take a look at the top four categories.

Fresh Fruits, Berries, and Vegetables – This is the foundation of any diet and about 25% of your food intake should consist of this category. By eating foods full of healthy vitamins, nutrients, and enzymes your body will be gaining the building blocks needed for a healthy life.

Cooked Fruits, Berries, Vegetables, and Whole Grains – When you cook using these natural ingredients, you are creating a healthy meal. Examples of whole grains would include rice, oatmeal, barley, wheat.

Fresh meats, raw nuts, dairy, natural fats – Use these to cook with the fruits, vegetables, and whole grains. Raw Nuts make a great snack. Only use natural fats like butter, olive oil, sesame oil, etc for cooking and salad dressings.

Frozen Basic Foods – We don't all live in climates where fresh berries or certain vegetables are available. If fresh isn't available, then frozen is the next best thing. That's true for meats as well.

If you'll build your healthy eating around these categories, you will have a hard time going wrong.

Don't believe the marketing that would have you believe that an artificial sweetener is better for you than raw sugar. I'll pick butter any day over an artificial spread made with chemical flavorings and hydrogenated oils! I lost over 120 pounds by eating natural foods! By eating foods coming from these four categories, the body moves to a healthy weight.

Avoid artificial "foods", because they don't support health. Natural foods help create a body that is energetic and strong. Foods that have been processed and no longer resemble their natural state detract from your health. It's that simple.

WEEK 2 DAY 4: *Journal*

This isn't a journey focused on denial, but instead opens new doors of opportunity and exciting options. Your food choices aren't limited but wide open to the vast variety that nature has provided! Thinking of these top four food categories, what are five foods that you love and can be included in this grouping?

Here are some examples: Salsa, Baked Potato, Grilled Steak, Fresh made BBQ, Fresh Pineapple, Homemade Apple Sauce, and many others.

1. _____   4. _____

2. _____   5. _____

3. _____

This eating plan isn't about depravation or denial… it's about making wise choices that support health! You're allowed to have fun, make your own choices, and design a food plan that works for you.

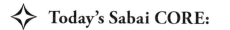 Today's Sabai CORE:

C – Cardio Movement   _____

O – Optimum Hydration   _____

R – Rest and Recovery   _____

E – Eat Healthy   _____

WEEK 2 DAY 5: *The Bottom Four*

Do not crave that ruler's delicacies, for that food is deceptive.
Proverbs 23:3

Let's take a look at the bottom four categories.

Healthy Restaurant Foods – It is quite possible to eat a healthy meal in a restaurant. Just make choices that build into your health. If you are at a meal for work and there are not a lot of great choices, then pick the healthiest, limit your portion and don't worry about it. You'll always control the portion and ingredients better at home than on the road. If you have a job that requires a lot of eating out, get really good at choosing the healthy meals. Many times an appetizer or salad is the perfect meal!

Prepared Foods – A popular choice for many is to pick up prepared foods at the grocery store, or prepackaged prepared meals from the grocer's freezer. Not only do you have less choice in the ingredients, but these have often been on the shelf for awhile before you ever get them. Remember, you want your food giving health and vibrancy to you, not zapping it out of you!

Packaged Foods – I call packaged foods "dead" because there's no life left in them. All the life was processed out of it and that's why it can sit on the shelf for months. Even if the product is advertised as healthy, organic, or all natural, if it has been processed to sit on a shelf for months, it is junk food. These foods don't add to your health but detract from it. While it can be difficult to totally avoid this category, it should only be a small portion of your food intake.

Splurge – This is a small category, but a fun one! This is where chocolate resides. I decided that when I'm going to splurge, it's going to be worth it. I'll have a small amount of a high quality treat. That naturally limits the amount and makes it more enjoyable. If it's chocolate, it's going to be a high cacao dark and if it's ice cream, it's going to have a small scoop of my favorite brand and flavor. When you are going to splurge, the idea is to savor a small portion rather than gorge.

By limiting these four categories, you're setting yourself up for success. Limiting doesn't mean eliminating, it means restricting how often and how much your food comes from these categories.

WEEK 2 DAY 5: *Journal*

I love the verse for today. It's really not the "delicacies" that we need but the basics that God has created for us. The more that food is processed and refined, it becomes like the ruler's delicacies. It tastes good but that taste is deceptive because it detracts from our health.

Being in the bottom four of our food pyramid doesn't mean that these foods aren't allowed, but instead that we make wise choices and limit these to a small percentage of the food that we eat. Consider what some foods are in these categories that you will "pass" on and ones that you will "choose".

Here is an example: Pass – Double Cheeseburger,
                        Choose –Salad with Grilled Salmon

	Pass	**Choose**
Restaurant Foods.	_____	_____
Prepared Foods	_____	_____
Packaged Foods	_____	_____
Splurge	_____	_____

You want to limit your intake of these food categories. You don't need to avoid them completely. For most of us, total avoidance is unrealistic and just sets us up for failure. Instead, set yourself up for success by making wise choices and setting limits!

✦ Today's Sabai CORE:

C – Cardio Movement   _____

O – Optimum Hydration   _____

R – Rest and Recovery   _____

E – Eat Healthy   _____

Week 2 Day 6: *Succeeding while "off-course"*

> *Now a great windstorm developed and the waves were breaking into the boat, so that the boat was nearly swamped. But he was in the stern, sleeping on a cushion. They woke him up and said to him, "Teacher, don't you care that we are about to die?" So he got up and rebuked the wind, and said to the sea, "Be quiet! Calm down!" Then the wind stopped, and it was dead calm. And he said to them, "Why are you cowardly? Do you still not have faith? Mark 4:37-40 (NET)*

Getting off course doesn't mean you've failed. It usually means that you need to make a small shift. One of the most common lies that we tell ourselves is that when we've eaten that cookie or some chocolate is that we've failed. The reality is that you can be achieving your goal while being "off-course" quite often during the journey.

Let me give you an example. Let's say that you're in New York City and heading to Los Angeles by car. Imagine a line pointing through the center of the car and extending in the direction you're going. During your 2500 mile journey, rarely does the direction of the car exactly align with your goal, Los Angeles. Instead, you are going that general direction during most of the time while not 100% on target.

What is your response to being off-course during that drive to Los Angeles? You don't throw the map on the floor and say "That's it, I give up. I can't believe I messed up already!" No. You don't quit just because you're off course. In fact, you realize that if you're heading west, you may occasionally head a bit north or south during the journey as well.

The same is true when you're gaining health. Eating that piece of chocolate cake at a birthday party doesn't mean that you've failed. I lost my weight while often off-course. Rarely did I have a "perfect" day, with the right amount of water, all healthy foods, a wonderful workout, and an eight hour night's sleep.

The goal is to have a majority of these going in the right direction. Do what's right and limit what's not.

Week 2 Day 6: *Journal*

As the waves crashed into the boat, the disciples were off course in several ways. Not only was the boat whipped around by the wind and not getting them where they wanted to go, but the disciples were gripped by fear, focusing on their peril. These were the same men who later took the message of Christ to the world! The moments of doubt and fear in the boat were not the end but part of the process.

Identify and describe two of the feelings that you've experienced most over the past two weeks.

1. _____

2. _____

Are these emotions empowering? If they are then keep doing what you're doing! If not, then change your focus! Disempowering emotions come from focusing on failures and frustrations rather than successes. They can also come from focusing on what you don't control, rather than what you can. What are two things that you've done great in the past thirteen days?

1. _____

2. _____

Focus on your successes and you'll achieve more success! What are the changes that you're most excited about seeing during these 12 weeks?

_____

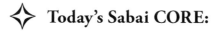 Today's Sabai CORE:

C – Cardio Movement   _____

O – Optimum Hydration   _____

R – Rest and Recovery   _____

E – Eat Healthy   _____

Week 2 Day 7: *Excuse or Motivation?*

> *Then the one who had received the one talent came and said, 'Sir, I knew that you were a hard man, harvesting where you did not sow, and gathering where you did not scatter seed, so I was afraid, and I went and hid your talent in the ground. See, you have what is yours. Matthew 25:24-25 (NET)*

As a tall man who was badly out of shape, I often had back spasms. My knees had pain and my left knee was very weak ever since a knee surgery back in 1991. Not the usual recipe for a fitness focused triathlete!

In reality, we all have challenges. It's part of life. It's interesting that the same challenge that serves as an excuse for one person serves as a motivation for someone else. Let me give you an example:

Challenge: I'm 45 lbs overweight and my knees hurt.

That challenge can become an excuse, "My knees hurt so I'm not exercising today". That challenge can instead become a motivation, "My knees hurt because I keep putting this extra weight on them. I'm going to figure out an exercise program that helps me lose weight while taking care of my knees."

If we follow the excuse and decide not to exercise, we have doomed ourselves to a life with bad knees. If we instead use this challenge as a motivation for change, we'll lose the weight which puts excess pressure on the knees. In the process, we'll also strengthen muscles which help stabilize the knee!

I'm often amazed at the power of these choices in life. Two children from the same abusive father can lead very different lives based on how they use the past. One may decide to hurt others because he has been hurt. The other may choose to serve others and help those who've suffered abuse because he understands.

Excuses lead to failure. Turning challenges into motivation leads to success. Do you typically make excuses, or do you use the challenges to create your motivation for success?

Let your challenge drive you forward and leave the excuses behind!

WEEK 2 DAY 7: *Journal*

The servant in today's verses was full of excuses and blamed his failure on others. If you read further in Matthew, you'll notice that the same excuses that he used were the reasons for the other servants' successes! When you hear yourself give an excuse for why you cannot do something great, immediately restate it as a reason why you must.

What are your challenges and how can you use those challenges as motivation?

Challenge   Motivation

_____   _____

_____   _____

_____   _____

Sometimes you need to step back for a few minutes to notice what those challenges are. Take the time that you need to really consider how the same challenges can be used as motivation in your journey!

✦ Today's Sabai CORE:

C – Cardio Movement   _____

O – Optimum Hydration   _____

R – Rest and Recovery   _____

E – Eat Healthy   _____

Week 3 Day 1: *You won't get fat eating an apple*

The land produced vegetation – plants yielding seeds according to their kinds, and trees bearing fruit with seed in it according to their kinds. God saw that it was good. Genesis 1:12 (NET)

I remember once wondering how many calories an apple had. My Mom looked at me like I was crazy and said "You won't get fat eating an apple". You know, it's true!

In making a shift from being unhealthy to making healthy choices and losing the excess weight, I've thought often of her remark. During this journey of gaining health while losing weight, I didn't count calories. Instead I've started choosing healthy foods. A typical breakfast has been homemade granola with yogurt and fruit. Lunches are often salads with a bit of meat topping. Dinner has a meat, veggies, and a serving of potato, rice, or homemade bread. In between meals, snacks consist of healthy choices like a piece of fruit or some raw nuts.

I'm not saying that you shouldn't count calories, if that's what is working for you. The challenge is that it didn't work for me and was shifting my focus from what's most important.

A half cup of blueberries has more calories than a few jelly beans, but the blueberries will assist in your journey toward health while the jelly beans do not. The most important diet choice is to choose healthy foods. We've gotten so warped in our concept of what is healthy. Somehow a calorie-reduced processed snack food is advertised as a better choice than a natural, wholesome food. Diet soda is considered better than fresh juice. Don't believe it!

God made the foods we need to be healthy. We don't need a huge company to design high sodium, low calorie foods packed with chemicals and preservatives to lose weight. We need to eat the foods that God designed to give health.

You won't get fat eating an apple.

Week 3 Day 1: *Journal*

God has created great foods that support your body's health. What are some healthy foods that you love? These are foods that are natural and/or homemade and have not been processed.

Examples from my favorites include: Fresh pineapple, homemade apple sauce, leg of lamb, lentil soup, and raw almonds. Write down your favorites:

_____

_____

_____

List some unhealthy and processed foods that you're willing to "put to the side" as you're on this journey. After you've reached your goals, you can always decide to pick them up again, in moderation.

_____

_____

_____

You'll find that as you continue in this process, your eating will become healthier along the way. The foods that once looked so good will look like something you don't even want to put in your mouth. Fresh, wholesome foods will be what your body craves.

◈ Today's Sabai CORE:

C – Cardio Movement _____

O – Optimum Hydration _____

R – Rest and Recovery _____

E – Eat Healthy _____

Week 3 Day 2: *If... Then Statements*

But the centurion replied, "Lord, I am not worthy to have you come under my roof. Instead, just say the word and my servant will be healed. Matthew 8:8 (NET)

Many times we have "if / then" statements that guide our actions that we don't even acknowledge. Sometimes these rules serve us but many times they don't! Let me give some common examples:

- If I can't exercise at least an hour, then I might as well not exercise at all.
- If I eat one item outside my diet, then I've failed and might as well eat anything!
- If I don't lose weight for one week, then it's not working.

The problem with these "if / then" statements is that they are based on lies. The truth is that any amount of exercise is better than none, no one food item makes your diet fail, and you may have weeks when you don't lose weight but do gain health! Most people have told themselves one of the above statements at some point and the result isn't pretty.

The "if / then" statements can also be constructed in such a way that they serve you and help in your journey toward health. Here are some much better examples:

- If I can't exercise at least an hour, then I'm going to take full advantage of the 30 minutes I have!
- If I eat one item outside my diet, then it will be a choice that I made and I'll pay the price with some extra exercise.
- If I don't lose weight for one week, then I'll focus on the health I gained. I'll evaluate my Sabai CORE to ensure I'm on track. If so, then I'm good!

Let your "if / then" statements help you along!

WEEK 3 DAY 2: *Journal*

In today's verse, the centurion had a choice. He could have done like others and had Jesus come to perform a miracle or he could speak the truth and acknowledge Christ's power. He knew that **IF** Jesus would just speak the word **THEN** his servant would be healed. How powerful!

What is an "if / then" statement that you've used in the past? How can you rewrite it to help in your journey rather than hinder?

Old statement:

If _____,

then _____,

New statement:

If _____,

then _____,

Be conscious of the "if / then" statements that you use throughout the week. Chances are you have some that you tell yourself often and take you away from your goal. Consciously rewrite these statements during the week to encourage and strengthen you in your journey!

✦ Today's Sabai CORE:

C – Cardio Movement   _____

O – Optimum Hydration   _____

R – Rest and Recovery   _____

E – Eat Healthy   _____

Week 3 Day 3: *Live In Today!*

> *So then, do not worry about tomorrow, for tomorrow will worry about itself. Today has enough trouble of its own. Matthew 6:34 (NET)*

You're on a wonderful journey which will reconnect you with your body and your health. Enjoy the process rather than waiting for it to be finished. The goal isn't to arrive at a goal but to establish patterns of healthy living today that will sustain you for a lifetime!

Oops. I let it slip. The goal isn't to arrive at a goal. Gaining health is a process. At some point during this process you will finish losing weight because your body will find equilibrium between your Sabai CORE implementation and your body shape. If you're always focused on how great it will be "one day", then you're missing all the great days along the way!

As I was losing my weight, people would often ask what my "final goal weight" was. My reply was that I had no idea. I trust that my body knows what my ideal weight is. At some point, the weight loss portion of this journey will end but that is only a new beginning. I've enjoyed each part of the process.

Continually seek health through your habits and activities. Whether you are 20 or 70, and whether a reforming couch potato or a seasoned athlete, there is always a heightened sense of health and accomplishment to be achieved.

The point is to gain health, so rather than push through to an artificial goal weight and quit the process, spend your efforts learning to live well.

Enjoy the process and learn to love it!

WEEK 3 DAY 3: *Journal*

Rather than getting caught up in the "one day" mentality, focus on the "today" mindset. What are you going to do today to gain health? What is a choice you can make today to honor God? By focusing on today and the choices you need to make, you're focusing where you can actually make a change. That's power!

What are some wonderful moments that you've had already in your journey toward health? What is great about being in this process?

_____

_____

_____

Note the moments along the way when you learn something, meet a new friend at the gym, or see a new muscle. Live in today!

Be grateful for the gifts you've been given in this day and you'll gain more health and blessing as you move into your future.

✦ Today's Sabai CORE:

C – Cardio Movement   _____

O – Optimum Hydration   _____

R – Rest and Recovery   _____

E – Eat Healthy   _____

WEEK 3 DAY 4: *Snacking*

Jesus was going through the grain fields on a Sabbath, and his disciples picked some heads of wheat, rubbed them in their hands, and ate them. Luke 6:1 (NET)

One of the most important ways to support your journey to health is healthy snacking. Your body wasn't designed to run on two or three meals a day.

Imagine when people hunted and were farmers. Did they hunt and harvest and only eat at 6 pm for a large dinner? Did they starve themselves as they waited for mealtime, or did they snack on some of their find throughout the day?

It's much healthier to snack and keep your blood sugar levels stable. With the standard three meals a day, we experience massive highs and lows of our blood sugar throughout the day. That urgent sense of "having to eat" often comes from a sharp dip in blood sugar levels after your meal has been processed.

Snack often enough that you stay out of that frantic hunger zone. In the beginning of your journey to health, you may need to snack a couple of times between meals. As your journey progresses, your meals will become well balanced with vegetables, fruits, and whole grains. You will find that your blood sugar will be more stable and you may only snack once between meals.

What foods make good snacks? Natural, uncooked fruits, vegetables, and nuts are the best. Examples are carrot sticks, fresh apple slices and whole raw almonds. By eating snacks during the day, you stabilize your blood sugar and keep you from getting into that frantic "hunger zone". You'll be able to focus on your work and life's mission, rather than food.

Regular and healthy snacks are a great way of caring for your body. By developing healthy snacking, you're setting yourself up for success!

WEEK 3 DAY 4: *Journal*

I love the image of the disciples walking through the grain fields with Jesus, rubbing the heads of wheat and eating them. Some translations say that the grain was corn. It's a great picture though, isn't it?

Your snacking can be similar. By eating something natural and fresh, you're giving your body the building blocks for health. While I was writing this section, I got up and grabbed some raw almonds to munch.

One of the biggest marketing ploys of our day is 100 calorie packs of cookies, fried nuts, and crackers. My Grandma used to say not to waste money on junk. She wasn't talking about food but she sure could have been! I'd rather eat 150 calories of something healthy than 100 calories of junk, any day!

Jot down some of snacks that you ate often in the past and new snacks that you're replacing them with now.

Past Snack   New Snack

_____   _____

_____   _____

_____   _____

Since your body is the temple of the Holy Spirit (1 Corinthians 6:19), only put foods into it that are worthy of being in a temple!

◆ Today's Sabai CORE:

C – Cardio Movement   _____

O – Optimum Hydration   _____

R – Rest and Recovery   _____

E – Eat Healthy   _____

WEEK 3 DAY 5: *Time Moves On*

As Jesus looked at him, he felt love for him and said, "You lack one thing. Go, sell whatever you have and give the money to the poor, and you will have treasure in heaven. Then come, follow me." But at this statement, the man looked sad and went away sorrowful, for he was very rich. Mark 10:21-22 (NET)

Often, we don't rise to meet challenges because of the time, money, or effort it will take to finish the task. Here's a little secret:

Time moves on whether you decide to make the change or not!

I had a co-worker once who wished they were brave enough to leave their job and attend medical school. Being a doctor was their lifelong goal but it would take seven years of advanced schooling and their residency before they would achieve their goal. Thirteen years have passed since our conversation and I've often thought about how his life would be different if he had pursued his goal. He would be in his sixth year of practice as a physician, but instead he continues working in that original job.

Time will pass whether you accomplish your goals or not. Get clear on your goals and begin working toward their fulfillment. Life gets exciting when your dreams start becoming a reality!

In one year, you can be either of these:

1. Healthy and fit
2. Wishing that you were healthy and fit

The difference will depend on how you use this coming year. Use this year to accomplish your dreams and create the healthy, vibrant body that you were created to have. Don't waste another moment wishing for the future but take the concrete steps needed to create it!

Rise to the challenge and design your future!

Week 3 Day 5: *Journal*

The young rich man had a simple choice to make, keep his money or follow Christ. He chose the money. Life continued on and whatever happened to that man, he missed one of the most incredible opportunities of his life. If he had given the money to the poor and followed Christ, how different would his life have been?

You have a choice to live a life of rich foods and excess, or live a life of moderation and health. The coming years will be incredibly different based on the choices you make now.

You know that time will pass and you can affect the results that you get. What are three items that you will commit to accomplishing? What is the time frame you expect it will take to get there? For example, you may want to finish your college degree in the next two years, or start a business in the next six months, or run your first 5k three months from now!

Goal:_____   Time Frame: _____

Goal:_____   Time Frame: _____

Goal:_____   Time Frame: _____

Decide to make time work for you. Make a commitment to achieve the changes that are important in your life. Time will pass and it's a great feeling to get where you want to be in life and know that you made the tough choices and followed through!

✦ Today's Sabai CORE:

C – Cardio Movement   _____

O – Optimum Hydration   _____

R – Rest and Recovery   _____

E – Eat Healthy   _____

WEEK 3 DAY 6: *How much exercise?*

Then Peter took hold of him by the right hand and raised him up, and at once the man's feet and ankles were made strong. He jumped up, stood and began walking around, and he entered the temple courts with them, walking and leaping and praising God.
Acts 3:7-8 (NET)

How much exercise you do each day depends on where you are in your current fitness level. It also depends on how quickly you'd like to get to your long-term weight.

If you find that you're incredibly sore, add a few extra recovery days into your week. By exercising two days then taking a recovery day, you can give yourself some extra time get over the soreness. That would give you three recovery days spread through the week.

As your fitness improves, work toward only one recovery day each week. The other days can contain varied workouts depending on your current fitness level. If you're easily winded and any exercise is a challenge, consider two 15 minute blocks of exercise during different times in the day. After a couple of weeks, you'll be able to up the workout time.

When you can do more, consider adding a third block and going to 45 minutes on alternate days. Later, if you choose, move to a full hour. For those days when you want to do extra, feel free to exercise more!

Be thankful for your ability to move and exercise. Each time you are sore, acknowledge how that means your muscles are growing strong. Your body is responding to the exercise by increasing muscle strength. The same exercise today that makes you sore will soon be easy to accomplish.

Though I started with 15 to 30 minutes a day, by my third week of the implementing the Sabai CORE, I had worked up to an hour of exercise each day. On Saturdays, I take more time and often do an activity that is longer. Sundays is typically my rest day when I spend some extra time with the family and don't plan a workout.

Recovery will give your body a chance to rebuild muscles that have been challenged during the workouts.

Always do enough exercise to keep your forward momentum going!

WEEK 3 DAY 6: *Journal*

The beggar that Peter healed was thrilled to be able to physically move. He jumped, leaped, walked and praised God! Aren't you thankful that you have the ability to do the same? Let's thank God for our ability to workout, stretch, and grow in our fitness.

What are some healthy activities that you enjoy, or have enjoyed in the past? Choose some activities that you would like to do today, or sometime in the near future that you can plan!

_____

_____

_____

I love the image of the beggar jumping up in excitement. List some times that you've leapt for joy or played like a kid? I remember fun times at Disney with the family or running down the beach in sunny California. As you gain health, you'll find yourself enjoying more of these times of excitement and joy.

✦ Today's Sabai CORE:

C – Cardio Movement   _____

O – Optimum Hydration   _____

R – Rest and Recovery   _____

E – Eat Healthy   _____

Week 3 Day 7: *The Lymph System*

Therefore, since we have these promises, dear friends, let us cleanse ourselves from everything that could defile the body and the spirit, and thus accomplish holiness out of reverence for God.
2ⁿᵈ Corinthians 7:1 (NET)

We're all familiar with the circulatory system. The heart pumps oxygen rich blood through your arteries to be delivered to your tissues. Did you know that your body has an amazing system that works in parallel with the circulatory system? This system is called the lymph system.

Like your circulatory system, the lymph system is a system of ducts that are throughout your body. The lymph system helps fight disease and clean the debris from our tissues and flushes it from our system. Without the cleansing of the lymph system, toxins accumulate and increase our risk for cancer, sickness and disease.

Unlike the circulatory system, there is no central pump to move the lymph through your body. Instead, the lymph moves by a series of one-way valves to insure that the lymphocytes which fight disease are circulated.

What's the problem with this scenario? Well, if you're not moving the lymph doesn't flow!

In order for the lymph system to work properly and help your body ward off sickness and disease, you've got to move! When you walk, run, bike, swim and move your body, you're helping bathe your tissues in a fluid that helps you stay strong and healthy.

You've seen lymph fluid before. When you've had a burn and clear liquid fills the blister, that's lymph there to help begin the healing!

You may notice during the first few weeks of exercise that you have excess mucus. That is the result of your lymph system moving out the crud! Today, when you exercise, visualize the lymph that is now flowing smoothly throughout your body.

You gain health when you move!

WEEK 3 DAY 7: *Journal*

It is amazing how God has created our bodies to be self-cleansing. Without our body's ability to fight disease and get rid of the waste, we could not live. As your lymph system gets re-engaged you may notice some changes. Perhaps you've had mucus discharge as your body cleanses itself. After the initial phase of the lymph removing the built up toxins, you'll begin feeling healthy and strong.

Changes are occurring deep within your body. Thinking about the lesson today, what are some benefits of a healthy lymph system?

_____

_____

_____

Let me commend you for being diligent in completing your journal! You are learning lessons that will help you become your best. This is a personal journey and an incredibly important one. The lessons you learn will help others find their way!

✦ Today's Sabai CORE:

C – Cardio Movement _____

O – Optimum Hydration _____

R – Rest and Recovery _____

E – Eat Healthy _____

Week 4 Day 1: *No Joy, No Gain*

"Look, God is my deliverer! I will trust in him and not fear.
For the Lord gives me strength and protects me; he has become
my deliverer." Joyfully you will draw water from the springs of
deliverance. Isaiah 12:2-3 (NET)

Life is made for joy and as we lean into the strength and protection God gives us, we can joyfully draw water from the springs of His deliverance. There is a joy that comes from accomplishing our life's mission. Believe it or not, your workouts were made for joy as well! When I mentioned splurges earlier in this book, I mentioned chocolate, which I love. That shouldn't surprise you!

There is a myth that's been around for ages, "no pain, no gain". While that may work for those who love pain, it doesn't work for most people! The truth is "no joy, no gain." Gaining health is a joyful experience. If the experience is painful, something is wrong.

Years ago, I heard the great endurance athlete Stu Mittleman, discuss running. He said that you should always be able to sing. What? Able to sing? Yes! When you are trying to catch your breath, you are in an anaerobic state and are burning the limited sugar in your muscles instead of fat. When your body burns sugar as fuel, lactic acid builds up in your muscles. The lactic acid from an anaerobic workout creates sore aching muscles that hurt! There is a better way. By staying in an aerobic state, you burn fat and limit the lactic acid.

When you are doing your cardio, you should have enough breath to sing or carry on a conversation. That means that you are still in an aerobic state, which is fat burning! Aerobic workouts are to your body and you'll recover faster from them. Aerobic workouts will increase your base metabolism and will energize you throughout the day!

Workout at an intensity that is challenging, but you could always burst out with a song. In fact… go ahead and try it… they'll enjoy it at the gym! You'll be more successful in the long run if you find joy in the journey!

WEEK 4 DAY 1: *Journal*

Choose a song that you can use to sing as a test to see if you're in aerobic mode.

_____

What's a choice that you can make that will bring more joy to your workouts?

_____

This journey is about joy and reaching your potential in life. Whenever pain or frustrations sneak in, it's time to make an adjustment that brings you closer to your healthy goals!

God is our deliverer. In Him we can trust and not fear! On the following lines, write some of your thoughts about the emotions of this time. Are you fearful, joyous, sad, or excited? Why?

_____

_____

_____

◇ Today's Sabai CORE:

C – Cardio Movement   _____

O – Optimum Hydration   _____

R – Rest and Recovery   _____

E – Eat Healthy   _____

WEEK 4 DAY 2: *Sore becomes Strong*

However, the war was prolonged between the house of Saul and the house of David. David was becoming steadily stronger, while the house of Saul was becoming increasingly weaker. 2nd Samuel 3:1 (NET)

Ask any athlete, it's difficult to stay at the same athletic level. They're either getting stronger or getting weaker. The same is true with everyone else! As you are working out, you're gaining strength but you're also getting sore, aren't you?

Around the fourth week of my journey toward health, I looked over at my beautiful wife Cindy and said, "Will we always be this sore?"

Thankfully, I can tell you that the answer is no. As a few months passed, my body responded to the Sabai CORE with energy, clarity of thought, and enthusiasm for the day! Sore becomes strong! Your body will become stronger and the soreness will fade.

I spoke in the last lesson about lactic acid and how it creates aches and pain. There is huge acid buildup when we first start working out because of all the junk that needs to get cleared out of our system.

Drinking extra water during these weeks will help flush the by-products of the workouts and fat burning. Don't worry that the water will show up on the scale. When you are drinking adequate water, your body doesn't feel the need to retain it!

As the weeks and months move forward, you'll notice an increasing energy that is naturally available to you all day long. That sense of energy "on tap" is your metabolism kicking into a higher gear.

You will begin to finish workouts feeling more energized than when you began. You will look in the mirror and see a healthy and excited person looking back.

The initial soreness is part of the process of gaining health. As your body strengthens, that soreness is replaced with health and vitality!

WEEK 4 DAY 2: *Journal*

Your sore muscles will quickly become strong muscles. As time goes by, they develop their strength and the fat that once hid your inner muscles will melt away.

Are you feeling sore from your workouts? Which muscle groups and areas are you feeling it the most?

_____

_____

_____

Your body will reflect what you're eating and drinking. As you exercise, drink lots of water, and eat healthy foods, you'll notice a new sparkle in your eye and confidence in your movements.

You'll also gain flexibility and balance in ways that will amaze you. As you walk, you'll feel strong and confident. You are one of God's children! Shouldn't you feel like one?

◆ Today's Sabai CORE:

C – Cardio Movement _____

O – Optimum Hydration _____

R – Rest and Recovery _____

E – Eat Healthy _____

WEEK 4 DAY 3: *It's Not All Positive*

Then they brought to him a demon-possessed man who was blind and mute. Jesus healed him so that he could speak and see. All the crowds were amazed and said, "Could this one be the Son of David?" But when the Pharisees heard this they said, "He does not cast out demons except by the power of Beelzebul, the ruler of demons!" Matthew 12:22-24 (NET)

I tend to be a positive thinker. I see the possibilities and the good in situations. Unfortunately, that's not a universal trait.

During your journey to health, you'll meet many like-minded friends who share your new found enthusiasm for fitness. You will also come across resentment from others who have unsuccessfully tried to lose weight in the past.

As weight starts dropping, you'll be surprised at some comments you receive. Here are comments that I received while losing weight:

- You're trying to make me look bad, aren't you?
- Too bad it all comes back when you stop dieting.
- If you lose weight fast you won't keep it off.
- It's so much harder to lose weight at your age.
- My friend lost weight but now she's bigger than before.

The challenge is that these negative comments will often come from those who you love most! Your friends and family love you and your change can be scary for them. Will you still love them when you're fit and healthy? Will your changes mean less time for them? Will you love them if they're not fit?

You'll also receive many comments which are positive and supportive. Choose to listen to these and let them into your heart. What is your Father in heaven thinking of your efforts? What does He think of your pursuing Health With A Mission?

Let your friends and family know you love them and set an example for them to follow!

WEEK 4 DAY 3: *Journal*

Isn't it incredible that as Christ helped others, the Pharisees saw it as evil? Unfortunately, you'll hear from others during your healthy changes that somehow it's bad for you. Be loving and kind, but be firm as well. Christ immediately responded that "Every kingdom divided against itself is destroyed, and no town or house divided against itself will stand." Matthew 12:25.

What would your responses be to the following? Be loving in your answer, but stand firmly for the truth. This is the model that Christ set for us throughout His life.

You're trying to make me look bad, aren't you?

_____

Too bad it all comes back when you stop.

_____

If you lose weight fast you won't keep it off.

_____

It gets so much harder to lose weight at your age.

_____

My friend lost weight but now she's bigger than before.

_____

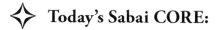 Today's Sabai CORE:

C – Cardio Movement

O – Optimum Hydration

R – Rest and Recovery

E – Eat Healthy

WEEK 4 DAY 4: *Replenishing Goals*

Later David defeated the Philistines and subdued them. He took Gath and its surrounding towns away from the Philistines. He defeated the Moabites; the Moabites became David's subjects and brought tribute. David defeated King Hadadezer of Zobah as far as Hamath, when he went to extend his authority to the Euphrates River. 1ˢᵗ Chronicles 18:1-3 (NET)

Humans are naturally goal oriented. We're designed to reach for our dreams and goals in life. Unfortunately, here's a scenario that's far too common:

1. An individual sets a goal weight to achieve.

2. Dieting is used to lose the weight.

3. Old habits are resumed when the goal is achieved and the weight is gained back, plus some.

Unfortunately, this is a scenario we've all seen or been part of in the past. Let's look at the issues that create this scenario.

Setting a goal weight: If the goal is a weight rather than health, then you'll seek any solutions to reach the goal, even if they hurt your body.

Dieting: Unless your weight loss is based creating healthy habits, then it will not be maintained.

The goal was the weight: When the weight loss was achieved they were "finished". They've achieved their goal. What's to drive them on to continue?

Healthy weight loss was my initial goal. Before that weight loss was completed I had set a goal of completing my first Olympic distance triathlon. Before that triathlon was completed, I set my next goal.

Set great goals and choose healthy ways of achieving them. By implementing the Sabai CORE, you will reach your weight goals over time.

Here's the secret, before you reach your goal, create the next one!

Week 4 Day 4: *Journal*

King David moved from one battle to the next. When he continued to keep a goal in front of him, he accomplished amazing things. When he decided to pamper himself and let others do the fighting, he used his free time to pursue another man's wife!

Having a great goal in front of you is a healthy way to live life. God designed us with the ability to achieve great things, when we have a goal in front of us. Without a goal... without something that's next, we tend to be directionless.

When setting ongoing goals, consider events that help you to continue your journey to health like learning to swim, running your first 5k road race, completing a sprint triathlon, hiking a trail, completing a metric century (100 km) on your bike, or attending a cooking school. As you gain health, what are some goals that you are setting?

_____

_____

_____

By continuing to set goals and participating in fitness oriented events, you are committing to remain on a healthy path in your life. That creates long term change!

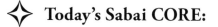 Today's Sabai CORE:

C – Cardio Movement _____

O – Optimum Hydration _____

R – Rest and Recovery _____

E – Eat Healthy _____

WEEK 4 DAY 5: *You Give the Kudos*

For we never appeared with flattering speech, as you know, nor with a pretext for greed – God is our witness – nor to seek glory from people, either from you or from others. 1ˢᵗ Thessalonians 2:5-6 (NET)

Where does your "glory" come from? Do you seek the approval of others for being so helpful, cooking a great dinner, or helping a friend? Are you thrilled to hear someone remark about the weight you've lost?

We all love kudos for a job well done and it's nice to hear people acknowledge that we're accomplishing our goals. While this is great to hear, it is not going to last over time. As you become strong and fit, your healthy body and fit lifestyle will become your identity in other people's eyes and the changes will become more subtle rather than so obvious. When that happens, the compliments from others can fade into a distant memory.

The lesson that we can take from this is that the kudos (compliments) should come from within. Unless you become the primary motivator of yourself, your progress will rely on the unpredictable feedback of others.

Many of us have been taught that it's not ok to be proud of ourselves. That is not healthy. We should always acknowledge and support the truth.

Some people ignore or marginalize their accomplishments. For example: "Yeah, I did the triathlon but came in 150th", or "I lost weight I never should have put on in the first place".

Part of this journey is learning to give yourself the kudos that you rightfully deserve. Being self critical is counterproductive and leads to failure rather than success. Be honest with yourself about what you achieve and the goals you attain. Reward yourself with a massage, a special meal out with your sweetheart, or a framed photo to commemorate the occasion.

Give yourself the kudos you deserve!

WEEK 4 DAY 5: *Journal*

The other day I wrote a list of all the things I'd accomplished over the past 12 months at work. I was amazed when I worked on the list and it kept getting longer and longer. It's really easy to think that you haven't accomplished very much when you focus on the short term. Over time, amazing things are accomplished.

For example, today you may have walked 30 minutes rather than your normal forty-five. It's natural to focus on the shorter workout rather than how when a month ago you may not have gotten off the couch! Sometimes I'm frustrated because I didn't run as fast as I want to, but when I look back, I am amazed and proud of my progress.

List some of your accomplishments over the past month. Give yourself the kudos that you deserve for the changes you're implementing and the decisions you've made.

1. _____

2. _____

3. _____

By giving yourself the kudos for working out when you don't feel like it, giving yourself the rest that you need, or eating healthy while at a friend's dinner party, you are setting yourself up for a healthy life that's fun as well!

◆ Today's Sabai CORE:

C – Cardio Movement _____

O – Optimum Hydration _____

R – Rest and Recovery _____

E – Eat Healthy _____

WEEK 4 DAY 6: *The Expert on You*

By wisdom a house is built, and through understanding it is established; by knowledge its rooms are filled with all kinds of precious and pleasing treasures. Proverbs 24:3-4 (NET)

You are the world's foremost expert on you!

So many times we look to others to be the expert on what we should eat, how we should exercise, and every other aspect of our life. This puts experts in the wrong role. We should use experts to help us learn more but not put the responsibility for our health in their hands. I am here to help support you and teach you. My goal is to help you design a system that fits YOU!

Why would you relegate our health to another person when you are the only person with all the facts? You know what you like and dislike. You know what makes you feel healthy or lethargic. You know what motivates you and what is not motivating!

The responsibility for health is yours! You are responsible for the choices and who to listen to. You are responsible for the activities of your day and the food that you're eating.

Throughout the day, your brain sends signals regarding how things are working. Are you tired or energized? Are you hungry or full? Learn to listen to your body's signals, interpret them wisely and use this information to make wise decisions for your health.

You have more information available to make wise decisions than anyone else ever will. Let the "experts" to help you make the best decisions. Don't ask them to make the decisions for you! Develop your knowledge, and then use your knowledge to make decisions that support health.

You are the expert on you!

WEEK 4 DAY 6: *Journal*

Knowledge from others is helpful, if you apply it with wisdom to your life. This book is knowledge that I've learned and am teaching you. The responsibility remains with you. You are the one that knows yourself better than anyone else does. Filter what others say, including me. Apply their suggestions to your life with wisdom.

Keep in mind the other person's perspective and motive as well. A surgeon will likely see surgery as the answer to your knee aches. A car salesman will likely see the most recent model of his dealership's line as the perfect car for you. Someone on a new fad diet is going to tell you it's the latest and greatest because it justifies what they're doing.

Are there some times that you've followed other's advice without really thinking through whether it's the best idea for you? Journal your thoughts:

_____

_____

_____

Be wise and understanding when building your health. Use what you learn to develop your skills and gifts.

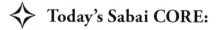 Today's Sabai CORE:

C – Cardio Movement   _____

O – Optimum Hydration   _____

R – Rest and Recovery   _____

E – Eat Healthy   _____

WEEK 4 DAY 7: *What's the Truth?*

These are the things you must do: Speak the truth, each of you, to one another. Practice true and righteous judgment in your courts. Zechariah 8:16 (NET)

We are sold lots of products throughout the day and bombarded with information. Some of this information is truth and some is lies. When writing this lesson, it was difficult to write the word "lies" because it sounds so strong! Wouldn't another word that is less harsh be better? No. The truth is that false information presented as true is accurately described as a lie.

Is it true that eating snack packs with 100 calories of junk will make you healthy? No. Eating foods that God created which are packed with natural vitamins, minerals, and naturally occurring calories will make you healthy.

Is it true that eating lots of artificial sweeteners and scientifically engineered diet products help you gain health? No. Your body has to work hard to get rid of all these artificial products. The truth is that the more you eat natural foods, with natural sugars, the more you cleanse your body from the artificial.

Is it true that the machine sold on late night television will be the answer to all your fitness problems? No. Fitness isn't found in a machine but in a mindset. There are many people in the world who are incredibly fit and have no access to expensive equipment.

Always answer a lie with the truth. Lies are like junk food for your ears. They may sound good but they take you in a negative direction.

Whenever you hear a lie, do not let it take hold in your mind and heart; instead, acknowledge that it is a lie and state the truth. For example, you read that a new diet pill stops fat from being absorbed by your body. Feel free to say out loud, "That doesn't sound healthy!" If I'm eating healthy foods, they have healthy fats like omega-3 that my body needs to be healthy. Always answer a lie with the truth.

In the truth, you'll find health.

WEEK 4 DAY 7: *Journal*

Identify some lies about health or dieting that you've heard.

_____

_____

_____

How can you answer those lies with the truth?

_____

_____

_____

The truth will take you closer to your health while lies will take you further away. Learn to evaluate the information that the media and advertising presents. Actively choose what information you are going to believe and decide what is not true.

Choose the truth and you'll find yourself gaining health!

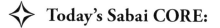 **Today's Sabai CORE:**

C – Cardio Movement   _____

O – Optimum Hydration   _____

R – Rest and Recovery   _____

E – Eat Healthy   _____

PART II: PEAKS AND VALLEYS

Every valley must be elevated, and every mountain and hill leveled. The rough terrain will become a level plain, the rugged landscape a wide valley. Isaiah 40:4 (NET)

Peaks and valleys are both part of a beautiful landscape. Embrace the difficult times as well as the emotional highs! As time goes on, the valleys will be less deep and the peaks more frequent. You'll live your days in health rather than based on your emotion.

Whether your day is at a peak or in a valley, appreciate the journey and the difference that each day brings. The peaks are wonderful and a great time for reflection and appreciation. The valleys are the times that build strength and character.

During these coming weeks, elevate the valleys and level the mountains and hills by creating consistency of action. Develop a routine that builds health by integrating the Sabai CORE into your daily activities. As time goes by, this becomes natural rather than out of the ordinary.

Every time that you exercise when you don't feel like it, you build the "muscle" of consistency. It becomes easier and easier each time that you strengthen your resolve. Every time you choose healthy foods over dead foods, you create a pattern that serves your body well.

Acknowledge that there will be peaks and valleys. Choose prior to either what your action will be. Yesterday, I ran a half marathon through Greenville, SC. It was a hilly terrain, so for much of the race I was either flying downhill or painfully toughing out an uphill climb. I'd determined before the race that the goal was to continue one foot in front of the other without stopping. The process was the same whether easy or difficult.

You are already a third of the way through this 12 weeks. You have already built consistency through the ups and downs. Take heart during the tough days and celebrate the successes at the peaks!

4 Week Measurements:

Today's Date:___/___/___

Weight:_____

Get an accurate weight by using a quality scale. If you weigh more than your present scale can handle, then your local hospital or health care provider should be able to help you get your initial weight.

One mile speed:_____

Map out a one mile distance. Walk, jog, or run this distance at your best pace. Record the time.

Waist:_____

Record your waist size using a measuring tape or record your pant size.

Chest:_____

Record your chest size using a measuring tape or record your shirt size.

Take a photograph to record your look at 4 weeks

☐ Check the box when you've done this.

Write down other measurements you'd like to record: (example: bust, thigh, arm, bench press, anything you want!)

_____

What are some positive differences you're seeing after the first 4 weeks?

_____

_____

_____

Week 5 Day 1: *Friends Along the Way*

As iron sharpens iron, so a person sharpens his friend. Proverbs 27:17 (NET)

In the first full month of this journey, I was visiting the states and working out in a local gym. I'd been proud of the progress I was making and was enjoying having a gym full of equipment available for exercise.

On this particular day though, nothing was working. My dream workouts on wonderful equipment were becoming nightmares. I was tired and frustrated. After 10 minutes on the elliptical trainer, I quit and sat down on a nearby weight bench.

That's when Paul came over and said hi. He and his wife had noticed my intensity on the elliptical trainer the day before and he thought he'd introduce himself. Within minutes, we were chatting like long lost friends. A few days later we scheduled a workout together.

In the time since that meeting, we've encouraged each other through Facebook messages, reading each other's fitness blogs, and emailing. The other day we were both doing swim workouts at the gym. I swam faster than I'd ever swum before!

Each like-minded friend that you meet during your journey will play a part in your continued success. By developing a small group of three or four friends that are on a similar journey, you'll each build up and encourage the others.

Like your Mom told you, pick your friends well. You want to surround yourself with others who are as committed (or more) to health as you are!

A group of friends is stronger than an individual.

Week 5 Day 1: *Journal*

As today's verse notes, your friends can help make you better. They can support and encourage you. They can also challenge you to improve. You may find that other friends are not interested in helping your journey to health. There can be a lot of reasons including pain from past experiences, people who left them after making life changes, or just fear that this will take you away from them.

Some friends will be your biggest cheerleaders and want to run a 5k with you. Share this part of your life with these friends. Thank them for their encouragement and take them up on the offer of the 5k. You'll find your life change in some wonderful ways!

Who are some people that you've met or know that will support you in your journey?

_____

_____

Who could you ask to do some workouts, a run, or a bike ride with?

_____

Spend some extra time with those friends that help you get healthy. If a friend seems to be sabotaging your efforts by buying you donuts, baking you a cake (when it's not your birthday) or ordering extra cheesy nachos for you, it's time to have a talk with them. See if you can get down to the root cause and talk it out. Seek the Holy Spirit's discernment about where to spend your time.

✦ Today's Sabai CORE:

C – Cardio Movement   _____

O – Optimum Hydration   _____

R – Rest and Recovery   _____

E – Eat Healthy   _____

Week 5 Day 2: *Setting Milestones*

Guide me into your truth and teach me. For you are the God who delivers me; on you I rely all day long. Psalms 25:5 (NET)

During your journey to health, it's easy to lose perspective on how far you've come. As you learn the truth and begin applying those lessons to your life, it's easy to forget where you once were.

Set milestones along that way that help you track your progress. An example of a milestone is the second set of measurements that you just recorded. One day, in the near future, you'll look back on these measurements with amazement. As you continue along your journey, these milestones will be an important reminder of where you once were.

Sometimes people avoid milestones, as they want to leave the past behind and pretend it never happened. That's not healthy, as it negates a part of who you are and what your experience has been.

Take photos along the way and you'll be amazed by the changes when you lay the photos side by side. Your journey is taken in small steps but big progress is made over time.

The difficulty is acknowledging the progress from within our own skin. It seems at any given moment that we haven't gotten very far, until we look back and see the milestones that we have set along the way.

This morning while cycling, I was listening to a Jennifer Lopez song "Jennifer From the Block" that states, "No matter where I go, I know where I came from". I expect that has helped her remain grounded as a successful music artist. Throughout your life, acknowledge your past challenges and the work it took to overcome them! Remember where you came from.

People without milestones never notice their process and eventually stop making any. Milestones help you maintain a healthy perspective and appreciate the progress you've made.

Set milestones along the way!

Week 5 Day 2: *Journal*

What are some milestones you plan to record along the way? What are events that you can capture with photographs or journaling?

Examples might be your first 5k run or playing with the grandchildren at the beach.

_____

_____

_____

By setting milestones to mark your path, you're also providing a guide for others to follow. Remember that often those following your path will be those that you love most!

My children now run triathlons themselves and will say after dinner, "let's go for a run!" What a blessing it is when our healthy lifestyle is emulated by those we love.

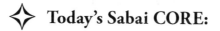 **Today's Sabai CORE:**

C – Cardio Movement   _____

O – Optimum Hydration   _____

R – Rest and Recovery   _____

E – Eat Healthy   _____

WEEK 5 DAY 3: *Get Back to Nature*

For the Lord is a great God, a great king who is superior to all gods. The depths of the earth are in his hand, and the mountain peaks belong to him. The sea is his, for he made it. His hands formed the dry land. Come! Let's bow down and worship! Let's kneel before the Lord, our creator! Psalms 95:3-6 (NET)

In a typical day, many Americans will move by car from their home to their office building. Then they return back home with a stop at a store or restaurant along the way. Each location is climate controlled and sealed off from nature.

There's something wrong with this picture.

In this journey, we've learned to rely on the foods that God made for us and move away from all the processed foods that man has made. In a similar way, we can begin spending time in God's creation rather than the whole day within man's structures and machines.

As you have begun daily exercise, perhaps you're already outside in nature more. That's great! Part of gaining health is getting more connected with the world that we were created to enjoy. When we spend our day secluded from nature, we're cutting ourselves off from one of God's most precious gifts.

This past weekend, my family and I headed out of town into the mountains. We spent an evening at a resort and took advantage of that opportunity to walk, swim, and play outdoors. What a blessing!

You don't need a gym membership to get healthy. Spend time outdoors walking, hiking, cycling, running, rollerblading, playing soccer, or any other activity that's going to let you get back in nature. Picnics with friends and outdoor concerts are a great way to connect with friends while spending time outdoors.

Enjoy the nature that God made and become part of it again. Feel the crinkle of leaves under your foot, the brisk air of fall and the radiant sunshine of summer.

Spend time in nature and be part of it!

WEEK 5 DAY 3: *Journal*

Consider today's verses and the majesty of God's creation. Three of my favorites are Edisto Island, SC, the mountains of Northern Thailand, and Northeast Harbor, Maine. What are your three favorite places that God has made? Where do you love to spend time outdoors?

1. _____

2. _____

3. _____

What are some ways that you get outdoors and exercise?

_____

_____

How will you add more time outdoors to your daily routine?

_____

_____

By getting outdoors and enjoying nature you are gaining health. Gyms and indoor activities are great but nothing compares to the great outdoors!

✦ Today's Sabai CORE:

C – Cardio Movement _____

O – Optimum Hydration _____

R – Rest and Recovery _____

E – Eat Healthy _____

WEEK 5 DAY 4: *Finish Strong!*

"Do you not know that all the runners in a stadium compete, but only one receives the prize? So run to win." 1ˢᵗ Corinthians 9:24 (NET)

Studies have shown that during world record setting performances, the athletes run the second half of the race is slightly faster than the first half.

Why is this true and how does it apply to you? There is efficiency in movement. By beginning at a slightly slower speed and increasing speed during the event, the athlete is tapping the momentum already created and feeding into that momentum during the event. It also means they have managed their energy supplies to allow a strong finish.

It applies to you because you are either an athlete or becoming one! As someone who works out regularly, you're an athlete in training. Use that training to develop your skill and improves your speed, stamina, reflexes, and endurance.

Take running for example. The least efficient part of the run is the beginning. You're developing a stride, setting a pace, adjusting your breathing, and getting into a rhythm. By building speed during the run, you are taking advantage of the work that has already been done and building on it.

By spending 40% of your effort on the first half of your workout and 60% of your effort on the last half, you'll finish strong and powerful. Take advantage of the momentum that you develop throughout the exercise and show yourself the possibilities during the second half. It's during these peak times that you'll surprise yourself by going farther or faster than ever before.

When you began this journey toward health, everything may have been a struggle. What do I eat? What exercise can I do today? It's taken awhile to develop your stride and a routine incorporating the Sabai CORE into your life. Now that you have that stride, push into it and enjoy the momentum.

Build into your work and finish strong!

WEEK 5 DAY 4: *Journal*

Running strong as you are in the midst of the race is a great sign. Are you running strong as we enter week 5 day 4? Now is a great time to take a deep breath, recommit, and plan your strong completion of this 12 week program.

What is an example of when you finished something strong? An example: The course in college when I went from a C at mid-term to an A by the end of the course or the Bible study our men's group did last fall.

_____

_____

What is an example of when you finished weaker than you could have?

_____

What could have been done differently to change the finish?

_____

List two things that you'll do so that you will finish strong:

1. _____

2. _____

✦ Today's Sabai CORE:

C – Cardio Movement   _____

O – Optimum Hydration   _____

R – Rest and Recovery   _____

E – Eat Healthy   _____

Week 5 Day 5: *Twice as far*

Therefore, since we have been declared righteous by faith, we have peace with God through our Lord Jesus Christ, through whom we have also obtained access by faith into this grace in which we stand, and we rejoice in the hope of God's glory. Not only this, but we also rejoice in sufferings, knowing that suffering produces endurance, and endurance, character, and character, hope. Romans 5:1-4 (NET)

My friend Phil, who is an avid cyclist, once told me, "You can go twice as far as you think you can." After a quick brain scramble, I said something brilliant like "What?" Phil explained that our beliefs end up holding us back more than our physical capabilities.

During this journey, I've had many opportunities to prove Phil correct. When I began cycling, I built up from 5 mile rides to 12 mile distances. Then one weekend, about three months after beginning my journey to health, a Phil and a friend asked me to go for a ride with them. As we climbed into the hills of Thailand, I had no idea what was ahead.

After an exhausting and exhilarating ride, I arrived back home with 30 miles on my odometer! I was amazed that I'd doubled my usual distance. Now my belief shifted from being able to cycle 30 miles.

The next week was the New Year and Phil and I began talking about a 62 mile (100 kilometers) ride to celebrate the incoming January 1st in fitness. The ride was amazing and my beliefs shifted again.

While I haven't done a 100 mile ride yet, I expect I could and will one day. In fact, the cycle distance for the Ironman competition is 112 miles and the Ironman is on my list of goals!

Rather than encouraging all of you to begin endurance sports, I'm just letting you know that your limits are the ones you've set in your mind.

You can go twice as far as you think!

Week 5 Day 5: *Journal*

I love this verse and the way it applies to this process. We learn to rejoice in the struggle of the workouts because overcoming that struggle produces character, and character produces lasting change. It's the overcoming and becoming more than you ever imagined which creates the lasting change. You will soon realize that you are a healthy, strong person. This will become your identity!

When is a time when you were able to accomplish more than you'd previously considered possible? Example: the time I ran for three miles straight!

_____

_____

_____

Name one area where you will test your limits physically today or tomorrow:

_____

Continue to stretch your limits and prove to yourself that you are stronger than you thought. You've got abilities and capacity that are amazing!

✦ Today's Sabai CORE:

C – Cardio Movement _____

O – Optimum Hydration _____

R – Rest and Recovery _____

E – Eat Healthy _____

WEEK 5 DAY 6: *Live the Truth*

"You will know the truth, and the truth will set you free." John 8:32 (NET)

What an amazing statement and so applicable to this journey! Statements like "I don't have time to exercise" or "I have to watch this TV show" are lies. The truth is that everyone can have the time to exercise and no TV show is a necessity.

Back in week four, we talked about truth in advertising. In this lesson, I want to talk about what you say to yourself that no one else can hear. Do you encourage yourself and speak with the love that God has for you? Do you see the possibilities and acknowledge God's wonderful design in your life?

Turn on the truth meter and start seeing things as they really are. One of the best ways to do this is identifying your self-talk that is true and what is false.

For example, perhaps you tell yourself "I don't have time to exercise". That is inherently false. Think of examples of people who are busier than you but find time to exercise. It's a matter of priorities.

Did you find time to watch three hours of TV last week? Did you spend time playing on the internet? There are always possibilities for using your time more effectively and changing your priorities.

Here is some self-talk based on the truth:

- God designed my body with an incredible resilience.
- As I develop my health, I can help others even more.
- My living healthy is an important example for my family
- I am becoming an athlete (as you prepare for your first race).
- I am an athlete (as you run your first race).

Live the truth and the truth will set you free.

WEEK 5 DAY 6: *Journal*

Are there any lies that you've been "buying into"? Write them so that they are easily identified as lies from now on.

_____

_____

Replace the lies with the truth by writing out what's true. For example, the lie "I don't have time to exercise" could be replaced with the truth "I have time to do the priorities I've chosen in life".

_____

_____

This is one of the most powerful lessons that you will ever learn. By identifying lies quickly, you can replace lies with the truth.

Look again at John 8:32. The Holy Spirit gives you the ability to discern the truth. By focusing on and living the truth, you will be free!

✦ Today's Sabai CORE:

C – Cardio Movement   _____

O – Optimum Hydration   _____

R – Rest and Recovery   _____

E – Eat Healthy   _____

WEEK 5 DAY 7: *Alternative workouts*

And let us take thought of how to spur one another on to love and good works, not abandoning our own meetings, as some are in the habit of doing, but encouraging each other, and even more so because you see the day drawing near. Hebrews 10:24-25 (NET)

We're all creatures of habit and as time goes by, you'll work into a habit in your workout routines. It's great to consider alternative workouts for those times when your usual activities won't work.

When I began writing this book, I lived in Thailand. During part of the year it's rainy season. Let me tell you, biking is more challenging in the pouring rain. What if biking is on the workout plan for the day and the skies open? It's time to fall back on an alternative workout.

Tae Bo and other quality workout videos are an excellent alternative when the weather is bad. The weather's always good in the TV room and its even climate controlled! The Nintendo Wii has a system called "Fit" that lets you do yoga, calisthenics, and play games that give you an aerobic workout.

The Biggest Loser workout book has great workout plans called "circuit training" that uses dumbbells and Body for Life has workout plans using a weight machine.

If dinner comes and you haven't exercised yet, head out for a walk after dinner. You'll feel better that you didn't drop the exercise for the day, but kept your consistency high!

By deciding several "fall-back" options in advance, you are setting the stage for success. It is ok to adjust with the day and change your plans. If someone stands stiff and rigid, they are easy to knock over. If they are limber and flexible, they can stand strong. Your workout plans need to stay limber and flexible.

Have an alternative workout tucked away for that rainy day!

WEEK 5 DAY 7: *Journal*

Rather than abandoning a workout, have backup workouts planned. If you have a swim planned and the pool is closed, what's next? Encourage others who are doing this course. If you don't have a group, join us online at www. healthwithamission.com.

What are three alternative workouts that you can pre-plan and have available when your regular workouts won't work? Example: Tae Bo Cardio or a walk in the park.

1. _____

2. _____

3. _____

By having these alternatives tucked away and ready, you have a plan for the eventual day when your regular workout won't work. You're planning for success!

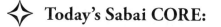 **Today's Sabai CORE:**

C – Cardio Movement   _____

O – Optimum Hydration   _____

R – Rest and Recovery   _____

E – Eat Healthy   _____

WEEK 6 DAY 1: *Small percentage differences*

> *"The one who is faithful in a very little is also faithful in much, and the one who is dishonest in a very little is also dishonest in much." Luke 16:10 (NET)*

Jim Collins, author of "Good to Great", notes that the difference between good companies and great companies is often a small shift that makes the big difference.

In baseball, a few percentage points can mean the difference between a multi-million dollar salary and the end of a career.

If you cut out a daily soda from your diet, which is a small percentage change in your total daily calories, you'll drop your calorie intake equivalent to 15 lbs of body fat per year!

Maybe a soda is too obvious, as most of us dropped sugar filled sodas at week one. Perhaps you've started this journey by doing 45 minute workouts. By upping the workout to 50 minutes, you've made a small shift that will make a difference by giving you an extra 125 minutes of exercise per month. That's like getting in a few extra days of workouts!

These small shifts are particularly important when we're feeling "stuck". Often we think we need to make big shifts when only small adjustments are needed.

The big shift was picking up this book and starting a new path. The small shifts are just as important!

Here are some examples of small shifts that make a big difference:

- Reducing portion size by 10%.
- Adding an after dinner walk each day.
- Packing a healthy lunch each day rather than eating out.
- Parking at the far side of the employee parking lot.

Next time you need to make an adjustment, consider the small shift that will get you there.

WEEK 6 DAY 1: *Journal*

Being faithful in the small things doesn't mean that you have to be perfect. It means that you don't take shortcuts. There will still be mistakes and areas where you can improve, but the dedication to mastering those small areas will pay large dividends!

What are three small changes that you can make that will get you closer to your goal?

1. _____

2. _____

3. _____

Implement these small shifts over the coming week and begin noticing the difference in moving from good to great. Small changes make all the difference!

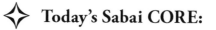 **Today's Sabai CORE:**

C – Cardio Movement   _____

O – Optimum Hydration   _____

R – Rest and Recovery   _____

E – Eat Healthy   _____

WEEK 6 DAY 2: *Everybody's got issues*

All have sinned and fall short of the glory of God. Romans 3:23 (NET)

My wife, Cindy, used to work with a nurse who would say, "Everybody's got issues." It's true! While you've got "issues" that you're working on, so do others. Just don't let their issues become yours.

In the first month of my journey, I visited a friend of mine. He had, like me, put on some pounds and settled into a lethargic lifestyle. My interest in losing my excess weight and gaining health challenged him to reconsider his position on the couch.

As he was heading to work one day, he asked what I'd be doing. "Going for a run on the beach", I responded. He quickly replied that "Running is terrible for your knees". I was disheartened. It was such a shift from how I had been feeling, I stopped for a minute to think. I remembered then that he was committed to avoiding fitness rather than embracing it.

Why would I take advice from someone who won't exercise? Why would I assign weight to his counsel? Be wise regarding who you accept counsel from.

There are a lot of reasons that people give advice. Some are helpful while some are not. Consider these examples:

- They are an expert and want to share what they've learned.
- They want to help you.
- They don't understand the subject but want to pretend what they do.
- They want to appear smart.

If an experienced athlete gives you advice on improving your freestyle swim stroke, feel free to take it. Excellent advice from experts actively engaged in their area of knowledge is a gift!

On the other hand, if an unhealthy friend gives you advice on why you're training too hard, feel free to leave that advice "on the table". Remember, everybody's got issues.

Just don't make their issues yours.

Week 6 Day 2: *Journal*

What is some fitness advice that you should "leave on the table"? Perhaps it comes from people with their own issues.

_____

_____

_____

Whose counsel would you consider and welcome in your journey?

_____

_____

_____

You'll get advice almost every day about health and weight loss. Evaluate the information, how much experience it's based on, and the health of the person dispensing advice.

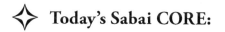 **Today's Sabai CORE:**

C – Cardio Movement   _____

O – Optimum Hydration   _____

R – Rest and Recovery   _____

E – Eat Healthy   _____

Week 6 Day 3: *Say what you mean*

His disciples said, "Look, now you are speaking plainly and not in obscure figures of speech! Now we know that you know everything and do not need anyone to ask you anything. Because of this, we believe that you have come from God." John 16:29-30 (NET)

I've got children and sometimes they will say something like "It would be nice to go to Antony's Italian sometime." My answer goes something like, "Yes, it would. We should do that sometime." They'll look surprised as they believe I didn't grasp their meaning. I'll talk to the children about stating what they want. What they really meant was, "Can we go Antony's for lunch today?"

If you won't tell others what you want or need, you will often be disappointed. Unbelievably, most people don't ask for what they want!

In restaurants, do you ask for what you really want? Perhaps you'd really like fresh steamed vegetables rather than mashed potatoes and gravy. Do you ask them for the substitution?

I've worked with my children and myself, in making sure that we ask for what we want clearly. People generally want to please and help others. If you let them know what you need, many will go out of their way to help you out!

Perhaps you're working with a personal trainer who is focused on your developing a weight lifting program and you're more interested in figuring out the treadmill first. Do you make your interests clear and does the trainer know your goals?

You've got to be clear about what you want and ask for exactly that. Otherwise you will live in constant disappointment that you're not getting the support and resources you need.

Say what you mean and ask for what you want!

WEEK 6 DAY 3: *Journal*

Here are some examples of not saying what you want: "It would be nice to go to a restaurant with some healthy choices" or "I had really wanted to workout today."

Instead, you could say: "Let's go to Inergy for dinner, they have some great healthy meals" or "Let's go shopping at 11, that way I can get my workout in now."

Give an example of a time when you didn't really ask for what you wanted?

_____

_____

_____

How will you word your new, clear, and direct request?

_____

_____

_____

In being clear about what you want, you give others the opportunity to succeed by meeting your request. Serve others by being direct and clear about what you want.

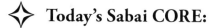 **Today's Sabai CORE:**

C – Cardio Movement _____

O – Optimum Hydration _____

R – Rest and Recovery _____

E – Eat Healthy _____

WEEK 6 DAY 4: *It's not a formula*

All the days ordained for me were recorded in your scroll before one of them came into existence. How difficult it is for me to fathom your thoughts about me, O God! How vast is their sum total! Psalms 139:16b-17 (NET)

Each pound of fat is 3500 calories, so if you reduce your calorie intake and increase your exercise so that you have a net deficit of 3500 calories, you'll lose a pound. Right? Wrong!

Ask anyone who's worked with people losing weight over time and they'll tell you that people are not machines and you cannot predict exactly how much weight will be lost.

The Biggest Loser TV show has shown this over and over again. After a wonderful week of dieting and hard work the scale will show no loss or a small loss. Why is this? Shouldn't it just come down to the math?

Your body is an incredibly complex system. Your body and mind are also dedicated to protecting you. As you're gaining health, your body needs to make a lot of adjustments. It's trying to decide what you're telling it now and creating set points along the way.

Rather than trying to force your body to make a change when it's resistant, a more effective strategy is to ask why your body is resisting the change. Remember, you're not in a weight loss competition with $250 K riding on the weekly scale.

Do you need more rest? More fresh fruit and veggies? More patience to let your body make the long-term shifts? Are you drinking adequate water? Have you eaten more processed or restaurant foods during the past week?

Finding these answers will help you make the long-term changes needed.

You are not a machine… It's not a formula… You are fearfully and wonderfully made.

WEEK 6 DAY 4: *Journal*

Is there a time when the scale did not show the weight that you expected to lose? What was your reaction?

_____

_____

_____

_____

How will you evaluate your results the next time they don't meet your expectations?

_____

_____

_____

_____

By choosing a realistic evaluation of the results, we create a platform for excellent questions and powerful answers that move us toward our goals.

✦ Today's Sabai CORE:

C – Cardio Movement _____

O – Optimum Hydration _____

R – Rest and Recovery _____

E – Eat Healthy _____

WEEK 6 DAY 5: *Stu's 85% rule*

A man was there who had a withered hand. And they asked Jesus, "Is it lawful to heal on the Sabbath?" so that they could accuse him. He said to them, "Would not any one of you, if he had one sheep that fell into a pit on the Sabbath, take hold of it and lift it out? How much more valuable is a person than a sheep! So it is lawful to do good on the Sabbath." Matthew 12:10-12 (NET)

In Stu Middleman's book, Slow Burn, he describes something called the 85% rule. Here's how it works…

Let's say that you've got a great plan for workouts. You've been following it faithfully over the past month. Thursday, you return home from work and are putting on your gym clothes when the phone rings. Your best friend from high school, who you haven't seen in 10 years is in town and wants to have dinner!

You've got several options:

- Tell her you've got other plans and can't get together tonight.
- Tell her that you can see her for a bit after your workout.
- Forget your workout and spend some time with your old friend.

You may be surprised, but my answer would be #3. Life happens and some things are more important than a single workout. If you become too rigid, then it works against health because it doesn't allow a natural balance in life.

This is where the 85% rule comes in. Work to do things well at least 85% of the time. Up to 15% of the time, allow for life to throw some curveballs or offer some special opportunities.

Have a hotdog with your son at a ballgame, and cake with your daughter on her birthday. That's the 15%.

Do what's right and honor your friends and family. Your health is given for you to help and serve others.

Joy is found in the balance between self and others.

Week 6 Day 5: *Journal*

Look at the verses for today. The law said that you could not work on the Sabbath, but Christ makes it clear that work is allowed if it is for good.

Often, in diets people get so fixated on rules when they rules are there to serve them, rather than them serve the rules. Why are you focused on gaining health? Perhaps so you can spend more time with your family, or so you can set a great example for others, or because you know God's design was for your health. Don't let your drive for health become unhealthy! Learn to dance with the changes that life throws your way, so that joy emanates from your movements. It's a lot more fun than being frustrated that the world isn't fitting into your plans!

How do you feel about Stu's 85% rule? Just because he has this rule doesn't mean that you need to adopt it. Rules are set up to serve us. What's your rule for the curveballs of life?

_____

_____

_____

By allowing some flexibility to meet life, we set ourselves up for success. Keep the percentage that you're doing high and you'll do great!

✦ Today's Sabai CORE:

C – Cardio Movement _____

O – Optimum Hydration _____

R – Rest and Recovery _____

E – Eat Healthy _____

WEEK 6 DAY 6: *Adjust your tack*

I look up toward the hills. From where does my help come? My help comes from the Lord, the Creator of heaven and earth! Psalms 121:1-2 (NET)

Sometimes small adjustments are needed to correct your direction and "adjust your tack".

When I was a child, growing up on the coast of Maine, there were free sailing lessons for the neighborhood kids during the summer. We'd all meet down at the harbor and get into groups of four and jump in the small sailboats. I loved sailing then and love it today. There's something about gliding gracefully over the water, making small adjustments in direction to take full advantage of the wind. Those small adjustments are called adjusting your tack. The tack is the direction the sailboat is heading and a slight adjustment of the rudder and tightening the sail can cause a major increase in speed.

As you start to develop momentum in gaining health, consider if there are any small adjustments that will make a big difference. One of the first adjustments was to increase the time I spent each day exercising. I found that I love the time out on the road cycling. By riding 20 minutes to work and back many days, I'd added 40 minutes to my workout time and the excess weight dropped off at an increased weight.

I adjusted my "tack". I was going to work anyway but just started to go by bicycle. While a small adjustment, it gave me an extra cardio workout, extra calorie burn, and an identity at work of someone who was serious about his health.

I've mentioned these small changes in several different lessons now because they are a key to your success. Life is unpredictable and things will change weekly, daily, or even hourly. Your success will hinge on how well you can adjust to the changes.

Sometime a small adjustment's all that's needed.

WEEK 6 DAY 6: *Journal*

How have you already "adjusted your tack" in the first month of this journey?

_____

_____

_____

Can you think of any adjustments that are currently called for? Remember, you may be right on course, so in that case, "no adjustments" is a great answer!

_____

_____

_____

Watching a motorcycle race recently, I was amazed by the constant and minute adjustments that the racers made. Adjustments are part of an active life!

✦ Today's Sabai CORE:

C – Cardio Movement   _____

O – Optimum Hydration   _____

R – Rest and Recovery   _____

E – Eat Healthy   _____

WEEK 6 DAY 7: *Muscles under the fat!*

Certainly you made my mind and heart; you wove me together in my mother's womb. I will give you thanks because your deeds are awesome and amazing. You knew me thoroughly; my bones were not hidden from you, when I was made in secret and sewed together in the depths of the earth. Your eyes saw me when I was inside the womb. Psalm 139:13-16a(NET)

Even when you can't see them yet, there are muscles under the fat. Can you lift 359 lbs? My legs did every day before I began my journey to health. Walking around with 359 lbs is bound to build some muscle! The challenge is that part of the weight was a layer of fat covering the powerful muscles that were moving the pounds.

If you've been carrying excess weight, you have muscles that skinny people only wish they had! One thing that I've enjoyed during this journey to health is uncovering the underlying muscle.

A few days ago, I was cycling back home from work and was stopped at a traffic light. When the light turned green, I pushed into the bike pedals, stood up off the saddle, and gripped the handlebars. As I powered through the intersection, I saw my forearms tensed with muscles defined and rock hard!

Unbelievable! My arms had gone from flabby to fit in a six month span and while my body wasn't yet "buff", my arms were.

Sometimes we get so focused on the outside rather than what's underneath. Quit focusing on the fat and instead focus on the strong heart and lungs underneath. Acknowledge the strong legs that have carried the weight. Acknowledge the heart that pumped blood through an extra two miles of capillaries in each pound of fat. Celebrate the body that is able to respond so quickly to the changes that you're making. Appreciate your body and what it's pulled you through.

Your body is amazing. During the coming months you'll see more and more of the beautiful body that has been covered up for too long.

The real you is in there.

WEEK 6 DAY 7: *Journal*

God designed you in intricate detail. He designed you with love and caring. As you uncover his wonderful design for your body, isn't it fun what you're finding? Can you imagine the smile on your savior's face as He sees you enjoying His creation?

What muscles are you most excited about developing and seeing? Why?

_____

_____

_____

What muscles may still be hidden but strong?

_____

_____

_____

Enjoy those glimpses you get of the strength and power you have in your muscles. Your heart is a muscle that contracts over 100,000 times a day... Talk about strong!

✦ Today's Sabai CORE:

C – Cardio Movement _____

O – Optimum Hydration _____

R – Rest and Recovery _____

E – Eat Healthy _____

WEEK 7 DAY 1: *Celebrate the changes*

"Now there were six stone water jars there for Jewish ceremonial washing, each holding twenty or thirty gallons. Jesus told the servants, "Fill the water jars with water." So they filled them up to the very top. Then he told them, "Now draw some out and take it to the head steward," and they did. When the head steward tasted the water that had been turned to wine, not knowing where it came from (though the servants who had drawn the water knew), he called the bridegroom and said to him, "Everyone serves the good wine first, and then the cheaper wine when the guests are drunk. You have kept the good wine until now!" Jesus did this as the first of his miraculous signs, in Cana of Galilee. In this way he revealed his glory, and his disciples believed in him." John 2:6-11 (NET)

When I was five or six months into my journey, I lay in bed one night and noticed something that I hadn't seen before. Right in the middle of my chest, there was this odd shape bulging up. Afraid that something was wrong, I showed the bump to my wife, who is a nurse, and she started laughing. "That's your sternum", she said.

My goodness! I had no idea that it looked like that! I hadn't seen it in such a long time.

In month nine of my journey, I put my hands to my sides and felt something odd. My belly wasn't soft but hard. After a bit of checking, I realized that I was feeling my "abs" for the first time. These are amazing times. Remember to celebrate them. Note them in your journal and mark the date. God continues his miracles today!

When I started my journey, there was a loop that I would ride on my bike. It felt like an adventure getting out of the neighborhood, past the lake and into the countryside. By the end of that ride, I'd cycled 5 miles. Six months later, I ran that same loop!

Every one of these changes and accomplishments are major! Tell the friends and family who support your journey. Write a blog so that you can share encouragement with others. Finish a 5k race and wear your t-shirt with pride!

Celebrate the changes along the way.

WEEK 7 DAY 1: *Journal*

What are some of the changes that you've noticed over these past two months?

_____

_____

Choose to celebrate these changes. Develop a deep appreciation for your body and the adjustments it's made along this journey.

How will you share these changes and accomplishments with others?

_____

By sharing what you've accomplished, you encourage others that are on a similar path. We need each other!

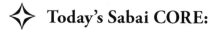 **Today's Sabai CORE:**

C – Cardio Movement   _____

O – Optimum Hydration   _____

R – Rest and Recovery   _____

E – Eat Healthy   _____

WEEK 7 DAY 2: *Learning Balance*

Certainly God is good to Israel, and to those whose motives are pure! But as for me, my feet almost slipped; my feet almost slid out from under me. Psalm 73:1b-2 (NET)

But I am continually with you; you hold my right hand. You guide me by your wise advice, and then you will lead me to a position of honor. Psalm 73:23-24 (NET)

I used to be scared to take a shower because I was worried that I would fall. Several times I almost did. I was so obese, I had a hard time turning around and I couldn't reach down very far without losing my balance. If I dropped the soap, I'd open another one because I couldn't reach it.

With the excess pounds off, my balance is completely changed! I can easily pick something off the floor, stand in the shower, and keep my balance while doing simple things like standing and putting on socks. Anyway, this lesson isn't about how balanced I've become even though that's cool. The ability to balance has just made me think about balance in other areas of life including this quest for health.

Exercise will help you become healthy unless you do so much that you don't give your body time to recover. Balance.

Healthy foods create healthy bodies unless the foods are consumed in excess. Balance.

Being active burns calories and sleep gives you the rest you need to be active. Balance.

Attaining and maintaining a healthy weight. Balance.

The secret to long-term success is realizing that the balance is a process, rather than a simple goal to be achieved. Balance is a series of continual adjustments.

Enjoy this process of learning balance.

WEEK 7 DAY 2: *Journal*

How long can you balance on one foot? What if the other foot is held higher than the opposite knee? Be sure to do this somewhere where you can grab something to regain your balance if necessary!

Your Time:_____

At week twelve, we'll do another one foot balance and see how much you've improved. You'll find yourself more balanced, strong, and flexible the longer you're on this journey.

Is there any other area of life where you'd love to develop balance? Write it down.

_____

If so, what is the first step you can make toward balance in that area?

_____

_____

_____

◆ Today's Sabai CORE:

C – Cardio Movement _____

O – Optimum Hydration _____

R – Rest and Recovery _____

E – Eat Healthy _____

WEEK 7 DAY 3: *You're worth it*

> *He himself bore our sins in his body on the tree, that we may cease from sinning and live for righteousness. By his wounds you were healed. For you were going astray like sheep but now you have turned back to the shepherd and guardian of your souls.*
> 1st *Peter 2:24-25 (NET)*

How much are you worth?

You are worth more than could be described. Ask someone on their deathbed what they would give to switch with you, in your current health. The richest individuals would give all they have and borrow more! Life is so valuable and you have been given a valuable gift.

One of our family's early decisions after beginning to gain health was whether to buy an elliptical trainer to give us an exercise option during the monsoon season in Thailand. It was a financial stretch for us and a family decision, as it meant we would have a light Christmas in terms of other presents. We decided to get it and have never regretted spending the money to support our health.

Have you ever noticed that nothing on the $1 menu looks very healthy? Many times it's going to cost more to buy a healthy meal than something quick and cheap. Our bodies weren't made to process junk. You're worth the price of healthy foods.

After 100 lbs of weight loss, it was not possible to wear my old shirts and pants. My wardrobe had to be replaced because I was looking like an orphan in everything baggy! I saw each new piece of clothing as a celebration of success.

Your savior gave His life for yours. How much is your life worth? Your life is precious and worth caring for. Great health is an excellent long term investment. Evaluate your purchases by how they support health. If they give you the resources to succeed, then they are of upmost importance.

You are worth it!

Week 7 Day 3: *Journal*

As a Christian, you have been adopted into God's family. You are a kid of the King! You are a unique creation, handcrafted by God. You have been given this gift of life and God has given you unique gifts.

You are valuable and loved.

Is there a time when you short changed yourself?

_____

What action can you take now to correct that? State something you will do this week because you're worth it.

_____

_____

_____

You are incredibly valuable and unique. As you progress down this path of health and fitness, you'll begin realizing just how incredible you are. You'll see your amazing body react and adjust to the demands.

◆ Today's Sabai CORE:

C – Cardio Movement   _____

O – Optimum Hydration   _____

R – Rest and Recovery   _____

E – Eat Healthy   _____

WEEK 7 DAY 4: *Forgiveness*

Therefore, as the elect of God, holy and dearly loved, clothe yourselves with a heart of mercy, kindness, humility, gentleness, and patience, bearing with one another and forgiving one another, if someone happens to have a complaint against anyone else. Just as the Lord has forgiven you, so you also forgive others. Colossians 3:12-13 (NET)

Imagine a person who is skinny and tall. As you get closer, you see that his skin has a yellowish tinge and has gotten leathery and aged beyond its years. As he smiles with stained teeth, he pulls out a cigarette, lights, and takes a deep drag into his lungs.

While he may have looked healthy at first glance, with a closer look, you've seen that inside, he is unhealthy. If you could see his lungs they would be blacked and gnarled from the years of abuse.

That's how it is with forgiveness. If anger and bitterness is kept inside, it becomes a black gnarled mess inside that eventually will show on the outside. Every time the issue is replayed in your mind, it's like taking a deep drag off a cigarette. It will destroy you inside and show up physically in ways you don't like.

Your journey to health will be lot more fun if the baggage of the past is left behind. Forgiveness is a gift that is powerful. It doesn't require an action on the other person's part; in fact, they don't even need to "deserve" forgiveness. Forgiving others is always powerful. Forgiving someone who has hurt you deeply or does not care about being forgiven is even more powerful. When you forgive "anyway", you've chosen health. You've done what's right even if they did what's wrong.

Jesus set the standard for forgiveness. He chose to forgive those who tormented him on the cross. Will you forgive those who've hurt you?

Gaining health is a process that gets rid of excess baggage. If something's unhealthy, drop it off and leave it behind.

Forgive and take a deep breath of crisp, clean air.

WEEK 7 DAY 4: *Journal*

Consider the verse for today. Forgive others as you have been forgiven. What's an example of a time you wronged someone else and they chose to forgive you?

_____

List anyone who you have not yet forgiven:

_____

_____

_____

If your list is blank, congratulations! If you have names on the list, then decide today whether you choose to forgive. Are there any actions you need to take? Often one of the best actions you can take is to pray for their health and for blessings in the other person's life.

_____

_____

_____

By choosing forgiveness, you've chosen to do what's right, even if you were wronged. That reflects strength and health!

◆ Today's Sabai CORE:

C – Cardio Movement   _____

O – Optimum Hydration   _____

R – Rest and Recovery   _____

E – Eat Healthy   _____

WEEK 7 DAY 5: *Consolidation times*

Therefore be very careful how you live – not as unwise but as wise, taking advantage of every opportunity, because the days are evil. For this reason do not be foolish, but be wise by understanding what the Lord's will is. Ephesians 5:15-17 (NET)

In your journey to health, weight loss happens in an uneven manner. At times the weight will come off quickly and at times the scale may not budge at all.

It's important to realize that you will have "consolidation weeks", or even a "consolidation month". After a sustained period of weight loss, your body often rebels and holds onto weight for a time. Relax… It's ok! Your body is doing what's natural and if you have more weight loss to go, it will begin dropping off again.

In general, weight loss occurs when you consume fewer calories than you're burning. You can decrease your calorie intake by controlling what you are eating and you can increase your calorie burn by exercising more. Your weight loss depends on many variables including fluid intake, salt intake, metabolism during non-exercise times, illness, etc.

Consolidation times are a wonderful time to review what you're doing. The Sabai CORE is critical to your long term success. Are you doing well in each area? Are you remaining committed to healthy foods? Is your exercise program adequate? Are you getting enough rest and recovery? Is your water intake appropriate? Make any needed adjustments.

Consolidation times can also be a special time of learning new distinctions and trying new things. Perhaps it's time to learn some new recipes or hike a new mountain trail. Talk with a trainer and set up a new weight routine. New exercises will create new changes in your body.

A plateau is fine for awhile, going downhill is not. As long as you are maintaining or gaining health, then you're on track. If the scale moves slowly, that's ok. Each plateau helps consolidate, or "lock in" the weight loss.

Consolidation creates permanence. That's a good thing!

Week 7 Day 5: *Journal*

Have you had a consolidation time yet? _____

How long did it last?_____

Was there something you did that helped weight loss resume?

_____

_____

Consolidation times are powerful and help you make the weight loss and changes permanent. Look at these as times when you are solidifying your health foundation. You don't have to rush it, but just keep evaluating if adjustments need to be made.

Remember that this journey is about gaining health. Gaining health is much more important than losing weight. If you're continuing to gain health, then any needed weight loss will happen in time.

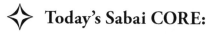 **Today's Sabai CORE:**

C – Cardio Movement _____

O – Optimum Hydration _____

R – Rest and Recovery _____

E – Eat Healthy _____

WEEK 7 DAY 6: *What's Your Identity?*

No, in all these things we have complete victory through him who loved us! For I am convinced that neither death, nor life, nor angels, nor heavenly rulers, nor things that are present, nor things to come, nor powers, nor height, nor depth, nor anything else in creation will be able to separate us from the love of God in Christ Jesus our Lord. Romans 8:37 -38 (NET)

Who are you? Our own self definition guides a lot of our actions and attitude. During this journey, work on a creating an identity shift.

Which of these describes you best?

1. A fat person trying to get healthy.

2. An overweight person working to regain control of their body.

3. A strong and healthy person committed to maintaining a healthy balance in life.

I would say that during the process of losing over 100 pounds, I moved through these identities progressively. Identity number one was me when I started this process. Within a few months I moved to the second identity and then later the third and most healthy identity.

As Christians, our identity should be based on God's design for our life rather than our shortcomings. If Peter's identity had been based in his denials of Christ, he could not have been the "rock" that the church was built on. Rather than define himself by his failures, he accepted the identity that Christ had of him.

If you define yourself as fat, overweight, a couch potato, etc, you will find yourself fulfilling this identity. Identity is a belief that is self-fulfilling. Base your identity on the truth! God designed you to be strong and healthy. Accept that identity!

Amy Grant saw herself as a world class music star before she ever was. I saw myself as a strong and healthy person committed to maintaining a healthy balance in life before I ever "got there". That identity is what helps you achieve it!

A healthy identity is based on God's design for your life. How has God designed you?

Week 7 Day 6: *Journal*

Write down how you see yourself physically:

_____

_____

_____

What is a more powerful self definition? How does God see you? What are the possibilities ahead by following His design?

_____

_____

_____

You will achieve your identity, whether it is destructive or empowering. A great identity is one based on God's vision for your life. Who has He designed you to be? What special gifts and talents do you have?

Choose an identity that serves your life and purpose.

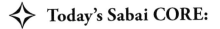 Today's Sabai CORE:

C – Cardio Movement   _____

O – Optimum Hydration   _____

R – Rest and Recovery   _____

E – Eat Healthy   _____

WEEK 7 DAY 7: *Be kind to yourself*

For as the skies are high above the earth, so his loyal love towers over his faithful followers. As far as the eastern horizon is from the west, so he removes the guilt of our rebellious actions from us. As a father has compassion on his children, so the Lord has compassion on his faithful followers. Psalm 103:11-13 (NET)

Do you find yourself denying yourself as a punishment for a missed goal? I know someone who decided that she wouldn't visit her daughter until she had lost 50 pounds! Once, I created a rule that I wouldn't grow a beard until I had gone below 300 pounds. How strange!

Evaluate these "punishments" against the question "Is this healthy and building into health?" The answer is no. Punishing yourself for your failings is a surefire way to create a miserable life. We all have times that are difficult and we're not doing what we should. We just want to acknowledge it, give ourselves some space, and then move into the future that we create!

Look at the verse today. God is compassionate to us and shouldn't we follow his lead? Sometimes people are less compassionate with themselves than with others. Rather than create an excuse for behavior, compassion can allow us to move beyond the past.

Find ways to be kind to yourself that create health and balance in your life. Here are some ideas that you can build on:

- Get a massage after a tough workout session.
- Build a fruit salad with all your favorite ingredients.
- Invite some friends over for a great meal.
- Visit a family member or friend who builds you up.
- Go rock climbing, mountain hiking, camping, fishing, surfing, to the beach, or anything that's active.

Acknowledge the hard work you've done to create health in your life. Give yourself rewards that build into that health. You deserve it!

Week 7 Day 7: *Journal*

Are there any punishments that you've given yourself to try to motivate yourself?

_____

_____

_____

What are some positive ways to create health and balance in your life? What are some rewards that you can give yourself?

_____

By shifting your focus from punishment to reward and encouragement, you'll begin seeking what's great in life. Build into others and build into yourself!

◆ Today's Sabai CORE:

C – Cardio Movement _____

O – Optimum Hydration _____

R – Rest and Recovery _____

E – Eat Healthy _____

WEEK 8 DAY 1: *Develop Your Cooking*

> *Do not destroy the work of God for the sake of food. For although all things are clean, it is wrong to cause anyone to stumble by what you eat. It is good not to eat meat or drink wine or to do anything that causes your brother to stumble. Romans 14:20-21 (NET)*

It difficult to control what you're eating if you don't prepare it yourself. If you've never learned to cook, it's time to learn! If you've always cooked, it's time to learn some new recipes.

I've always loved to cook and as you can imagine, many of my recipes were not the healthiest dishes. During this journey I've learned a lot of new recipes! Remember the inverted food pyramid and prepare meals that follow that format.

Strive to have fresh fruit and/or vegetables at each meal. You can make another portion of your meal cooked fresh fruits or vegetables, whole grains, and fresh cooked meat. Many of you will be cooking for others as well. Create meals that set the example for healthy living. This is a wonderful gift to give your family and loved ones.

Thankfully these days, there are a lot of great recipe sites on the internet. I post a lot of recipes on the site www.grouprecipes.com. There are many other cooking sites where you'll get useful ideas for variety in your foods. If your cooking skills are weak, consider taking a cooking school or offering to help a friend with her cooking. Another great site for encouragement and recipes is www.sparkrecipes.com. The recipes there include nutritional information.

If you have to eat out often for work meetings, become an expert in ordering healthy food at restaurants. A good calorie book will give you nutritional information for most major restaurants. You'll be surprised that some salads out can pack more than 1000 calories! Know what you're eating whether you're eating in or out.

A fun way to improve your cooking is to find a weekend cooking school or a friend who can help you learn. Having lots of foods that are tasty, fresh, and exactly what you love will help you in your journey.

Learn to cook healthy and treat yourself to a wonderful meal!

WEEK 8 DAY 1: *Journal*

What are some of your favorite healthy foods / recipes that you currently love?

_____

_____

_____

What are some healthy dishes that you'd love to be able to cook?

_____

Find one recipe on an online site that you will cook this week and write the name or web address below.

_____

By cooking and preparing your own food, you're taking control of what goes into your body. That's an incredibly important step in your journey to health!

✦ Today's Sabai CORE:

C – Cardio Movement _____

O – Optimum Hydration _____

R – Rest and Recovery _____

E – Eat Healthy _____

WEEK 8 DAY 2: *Built in rewards*

Look, the sovereign Lord comes as a victorious warrior; his military power establishes his rule. Look, his reward is with him; his prize goes before him. Like a shepherd he tends his flock; he gathers up the lambs with his arm; he carries them close to his heart; he leads the ewes along. Isaiah 40:10-11 (NET)

It's great to have rewards that keep you motivated and excited about your next step. Rather than falling into the trap of punishing yourself, create rewards that motivate. Rewarding yourself means choosing attainable goals and micro goals that are tangible and within reach and a reward that will follow the accomplishment.

Say you've got a bicycle that works but as you workout you become quite proficient at cycling and want to "step up your game". Setting an achievable goal that you'll accomplish before upgrading your bike can be a great way of keeping the motivation up. After finishing my first Ironman 70.3 in Augusta, Georgia, I knew I'd earned the bike upgrade.

Another example of reward can be a trip. I found a triathlon that started at Disney World, the Ironman 70.3 Florida. While I trained for the triathlon, I was also excited about it being a special time for the whole family. We saved and planned for this special trip and my brother's family joined us. My sister in law even ran the race with me! This trip was a grand celebration that we all enjoyed.

Any way that you can create these built in rewards will help you in accomplishing your goals. Let's break down why the prior example was so effective.

- I needed to exercise so signing up for a triathlon gave me an exciting goal that supports that exercise.

- Choosing a triathlon at Disney World made it a fun "destination" to be looking forward to.

- Involving the family made it a celebration for all of us. Rather than my exercise taking away from the family, it was creating fun times together.

Build in rewards celebrate your accomplishments!

WEEK 8 DAY 2: *Journal*

What is a goal that you have which you could develop a reward for? The reward can bless you, your family and your friends!

_____

Name a time when you accomplished something and there was an unexpected benefit.

_____

What is a dream goal that you'd love to achieve "one day" and what would the reward for that achievement be?

_____

Make your dreams a reality by planning them and rewarding yourself when you do something great! By lesson fifty, you are so much further ahead than many people have the discipline to achieve! Reward yourself with something healthy and fun!

✦ Today's Sabai CORE:

C – Cardio Movement   _____

O – Optimum Hydration   _____

R – Rest and Recovery   _____

E – Eat Healthy   _____

WEEK 8 DAY 3: *Chunk down your workout*

The diligent person will rule, but the slothful will become a slave. Proverbs 12:24 (NET)

Sometimes a workout can seem overwhelming. I find that, for me, the elliptical machine is particularly difficult. I like the challenge that it presents and the way sweat drips off me during the workout. I've found by "chunking down" the workout into smaller sections, it becomes much easier to accomplish. It's the same thing we did in an earlier lesson by breaking down an hour workout into four 15 minute sessions.

Here's how the elliptical workout breaks down for me:

- $1/20^{th}$ – 3 minutes
- $1/10^{th}$ – 6 minutes
- $1/8^{th}$ – 7:30 minutes
- $1/6^{th}$ – 10 minutes
- $1/5^{th}$ – 12 minutes
- $1/4^{th}$ – 15 minutes
- $1/3^{rd}$ – 20 minutes
- $2/5^{ths}$ – 24 minutes
- $1/2$ – 30 minutes
- $3/5^{th}$ – 36 minutes
- $2/3^{rd}$ – 40 minutes
- $4/5^{th}$ – 38 minutes
- $5/6^{th}$ – 50 minutes
- Done! – 60 minutes

By breaking it down this way, I achieve a micro-goal every few minutes. Whatever your exercise, there is a way to break it into manageable pieces. Sometimes an hour on the elliptical seems daunting but four 15 minute chunks are not quite as tough.

By design, a triathlon is divided into thirds and the athlete has a built in sense of accomplishment at each stage of the race. As the swimming finishes the triathlete looks forward to the bike. As the bike portion is completed, they know they're hitting the final run for the finish.

Whenever something looks tough, chunk it down!

WEEK 8 DAY 3: *Journal*

What are the workouts that you find the most challenging?

_____

Design a way to break those workouts into smaller chunks that you can acknowledge accomplishing along the way.

_____

_____

_____

By chunking down these tough workouts, you'll always be looking forward to accomplishing that next mini-goal. Many marathon runners count their race as 26 one mile runs with a .2 mile push at the end!

✦ Today's Sabai CORE:

C – Cardio Movement _____

O – Optimum Hydration _____

R – Rest and Recovery _____

E – Eat Healthy _____

WEEK 8 DAY 4: *Ask Better Questions*

"I, wisdom, live with prudence, and I find knowledge and discretion. The fear of the Lord is to hate evil; I hate arrogant pride and the evil way and perverse utterances. Counsel and sound wisdom belong to me; I possess understanding and might." ` Proverbs 8:12-14 (NET)

Avoid asking questions with no positive answer. Questions like "Why am I so fat?" only lead to bad answers like "Because I'm lazy" or "Because I've got a metabolism problem". Bad questions lead to bad answers.

Great questions, in contrast, lead to powerful answers. Examples are:

- What workout could I do tomorrow that would be a lot of fun?

- What are the healthiest choices on this menu?

- How can I add more exercise into my daily routine?

Many people have built bad questions into their lives. Days filled with "How can I be so stupid?" or "Why am I so weak?" create a life filled with frustration and sadness. I used to ask myself, "Why am I never good enough?" Let's look at why this question was so damaging:

1. It's based on an assumption that I am less than capable. I am fully capable because of Christ in me. The truth is that Christ's forgiveness, His power, and His direction lead me to amazing possibilities.

2. It looks for what's wrong rather than what's right. A question like "How can I accomplish this task God has before me?" is far more powerful as it creates a search for resources.

3. It discourages rather than encourages. Remember Philippians 4:8 states, "whatever is true, whatever is worthy of respect, whatever is just, whatever is pure, whatever is lovely, whatever is commendable, if something is excellent or praiseworthy, think about these things."

Your brain is a remarkable instrument. It is highly creative and made for problem solving. It will answer the questions that you pose, whether constructive or destructive.

Ask great questions whose answers take you where you want to go!

WEEK 8 DAY 4: *Journal*

What are some bad questions that lead to bad answers that you have asked yourself in the past?

_____

_____

_____

What are some empowering questions that you can replace them with any time those previous questions come to mind?

_____

_____

_____

By asking better questions, you create an environment where you are successful and the questions help you move toward fitness. When your mind asks a question, evaluate the power of that question before you answer!

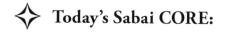 Today's Sabai CORE:

C – Cardio Movement   _____

O – Optimum Hydration   _____

R – Rest and Recovery   _____

E – Eat Healthy   _____

WEEK 8 DAY 5: *Whose Responsibility is it?*

So then whether we are alive or away, we make it our ambition to please him. For we must all appear before the judgment seat of Christ, so that each one may be paid back according to what he has done while in the body, whether good or evil. 2nd Corinthians 5:9-10 (NET)

Your health is your responsibility. While aspects may not always be under your control, your response to those issues is in your hands.

Others can provide resources and ideas, but it's your responsibility to implement them. How often have you excused an unhealthy meal with "that's where they wanted to eat"? Have you missed workouts because of others influence on your schedule? It is one thing to choose to miss a workout but you cannot allow others to decide what your priorities are. The responsibility is yours.

In this book, I've relayed the lessons that have helped me in my journey. It's your responsibility to apply these lessons to your life and find your own road. I can't do the journal for you or apply the lessons to your life! While our journeys can be similar, they will not be the same. With every decision you make, every change you implement, you are creating a path to health that is as individual as you are!

At times it's tempting to have a weight loss service send meals, or join some diet craze that promises an easy answer without your thought going into the process. It's your mental shifts that create permanent changes. Your answers won't come passively but only with active effort and pursuit.

There is an incredible power to accepting responsibility. You have choices and you have control. The success or failure rests on your shoulders. Move forward with that responsibility and make wise decisions.

Create your health plan that includes resources that you have chosen because they build into your body, making you stronger and fit. Success will be due to your tenacity and plan rather than someone else's fad diet of the day.

Your health is your responsibility.

WEEK 8 DAY 5: *Journal*

Are you ready to take responsibility for your health today? Write your "declaration of independence" from others and choose to be responsible for your health and fitness!

_____

_____

_____

_____

_____

_____

By choosing to assert your responsibility for your health, you've chosen to have authority and direction over your fitness level. Make decisions that drive you toward health and acknowledge your wise choices!

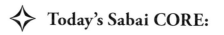 **Today's Sabai CORE:**

C – Cardio Movement _____

O – Optimum Hydration _____

R – Rest and Recovery _____

E – Eat Healthy _____

WEEK 8 DAY 6: *Shortcuts are Short Term*

> *But reject those myths fit only for the godless and gullible, and train yourself for godliness. For "physical exercise has some value, but godliness is valuable in every way. It holds promise for the present life and for the life to come." 1st Timothy 4:7-8 (NET)*

Extreme diets can help you lose weight but it's a short-term "fix". Without a long-term solution, we're back to our same problems as soon as the weight loss goal is reached or we quit the crazy diet.

Have you ever noticed that the people who chase the shortcuts are never fulfilled? Whether a "get rich quick" scheme or the latest fad diet, if any results are achieved, they are short-lived.

Here's the bigger issue, these shortcuts often exact a high price. While someone is benefitting, it often is not the person in need but the person doing the marketing!

By the time you've finished this book, you will have implemented the Sabai CORE for 12 weeks! You will have dug deep and dealt with the central issues that had you gaining weight. There's nothing shortcut about this book because it takes hard work and you create the answers!

The best way to effectively get where you want to go is to get directions. Find someone who's gone there and draw a map. That's what this book does. By working daily on the Sabai CORE, you're addressing the physical changes that need to be made. By working through the journal, you're addressing the mental shifts that are needed.

The truth is that the "long cut" is often the best answer. Doing things right the first time may not always be easy but the results are outstanding. There are so many examples of how true this is. Imagine that you're buying a piece of furniture that you want to pass down to your children. The quickly fabricated pieces won't last the test of time. The piece that was created by a craftsman with time and focus will last for centuries. Have you treated your health with short cuts or long cuts? Are you taking the time to "do it right"?

Focus on your long term destination and make the changes needed to arrive at your goal. Short term fads won't get you to your long term goal.

Commit to the changes needed to success long term!

WEEK 8 DAY 6: *Journal*

What are some shortcuts you've taken in the past that didn't take you to a long term solution?

_____

_____

_____

What is the long term solution that will get you there and keep you at a healthy weight?

_____

_____

_____

By choosing the long term solution, you're making a shift that will be life altering. It's these choices that change character and develop the traits of discipline, truth, and respect that serve you in all areas of life.

◆ Today's Sabai CORE:

C – Cardio Movement   _____

O – Optimum Hydration   _____

R – Rest and Recovery   _____

E – Eat Healthy   _____

Week 8 Day 7: *Diamonds and Stones*

Diamond: And I tell you that you are Peter, and on this rock I will build my church, and the gates of Hades will not overpower it. Matthew 16:18 (NET)

Stone: At that he began to curse, and he swore with an oath, "I do not know the man!" At that moment a rooster crowed. Then Peter remembered what Jesus had said: "Before the rooster crows, you will deny me three times." And he went outside and wept bitterly. Matthew 26:74-75 (NET)

Maybe the saying is "some days are diamond and some days are stones" but at times "weeks" is more accurate. After 25 weeks of losing weight consecutively, I had a week with a two pound gain. There was a "perfect storm" of issues that helped create the problem. Important guests arrived, I injured my knee while running, and I was tired and overextended. I needed a break.

After a weeklong rest, the scale showed an increase in weight! I thought I'd never gain weight again. I was wrong. At first, I was frustrated but after some thought I realized, it's ok to have a rough week.

Some weeks are diamonds and some weeks are stones.

While riding my bicycle and reflecting on the stone week that had passed, I was reminded of Microsoft. I'm a computer guy so stick with me, the analogy will make sense.

In June 1991, Microsoft stock plummeted over 32%. Investors second guessed themselves and wondered what they had done wrong. Many of them sold their stock. Those that have stayed the course since the company's inception have gained over 31000%!

Do you ever feel like you've had a week where your "stock" has plummeted 32%? It's easy in those times to forget those weeks and months where consistent improvements were made. It's not about a week, diamond or stone. It's about a path and continually working toward your fitness goals.

Long term goals are accomplished over time. By consistent action and continuing after a setback, you'll create a life that is a diamond!

Week 8 Day 7: *Journal*

What are some weeks that have been difficult in your journey over the past two months?

_____

_____

_____

Why did you decide to continue your journey rather than quitting?

_____

By choosing to continue, you develop the "muscles" of determination, wisdom, and courage. Acknowledge yourself when you choose to push through those difficult times!

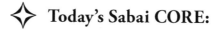 **Today's Sabai CORE:**

C – Cardio Movement _____

O – Optimum Hydration _____

R – Rest and Recovery _____

E – Eat Healthy _____

PART III: IDENTITY

For I am convinced that neither death, nor life, nor angels, nor heavenly rulers, nor things that are present, nor things to come, nor powers, nor height, nor depth, nor anything else in creation will be able to separate us from the love of God in Christ Jesus our Lord. Romans 8:38-29 (NET)

Wow! Here you are two months into your journey. You've discovered the Sabai CORE and incorporated these principles into your life. The goal is to make this lifestyle a natural part of who you are. During the next four weeks, you'll take a closer look at who you are and what created prior issues.

Consider these verses from Romans that speak about how loved you are. Nothing can separate you from the love of God and you are His child. Accept this love and move forward in full knowledge of it. You are a child of The King and were designed for a life full of excitement, adventure, and accomplishment.

Take a clear look at the issues and make a choice about who you are. During these next four weeks, we will explore your identity and give you choices for the future. Your identity is indeed a powerful force and you can design it for long term success!

8 WEEK MEASUREMENTS:

Date:___/___/___

Use a cloth tape measure to get the following measurements. Also get an accurate weight, so that we have these numbers for reference. Look back at your measurements when you started and note your differences!

Weight:_____

One mile or kilometer timed:_____

Waist:_____

Chest:_____

Any other measurements you'd like to take:

_____

_____

_____

What are some differences you're seeing after the first 8 weeks?

_____

_____

_____

Week 9 Day 1: *Work on Your Weakness*

> *But he said to me, "My grace is enough for you, for my power is made perfect in weakness." So then, I will boast most gladly about my weaknesses, so that the power of Christ may reside in me. Therefore I am content with weaknesses, with insults, with troubles, with persecutions and difficulties for the sake of Christ, for whenever I am weak, then I am strong. 2ⁿᵈ Corinthians 12:9-10 (NET)*

As I've been preparing for triathlons, I've really enjoyed learning the sport. I've worked on my running using Stu Middleman's book, "Slow Burn". I've been working on my swimming by reading Terry McLaughlin's "Total Immersion Swimming". I've also worked on my cycling by just doing it a lot!

I've also been reading Joe Friel, who's a wonderful triathlon coach and has written "The Triathlon Bible". He says that we should spend more time "working on our weakness" and that echoes throughout the triathlon community.

Isn't that a great idea to apply to life in general? What is your weakness? Consider the Sabai CORE. What are your strongest areas and which are your weakest?

Whatever your weakness, it is okay to have one. We all do! Choose your biggest weakness and make a focused effort to improve.

I realize that my weakest link in the triathlon is my swimming. Using the Total Immersion method, I'm working on that weakness and planning to turn that into strength. Within weeks my swimming improved to the point that I could easily swim the 750 meters of a sprint triathlon. During the next months, I worked on speed and becoming more fluid in my stroke.

In my Sabai CORE, the size of my food portion is my weakness and I've worked consciously on improving my portion control. My water intake was originally a weakness but today is one of the strongest parts of my Sabai CORE. By working on your weakness, you'll see exciting progress quickly.

What is your weakness? Work on it!

WEEK 9 DAY 1: *Journal*

What do you see as your weak areas?

_____

_____

_____

Write down some actions you will take to improve this area or find the resources you need to make progress?

_____

_____

_____

By choosing to work on your areas of weakness, you choose to control them rather than have them control you. By acknowledging weakness and developing those areas, what was once a weakness will become strength!

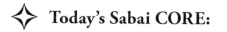 Today's Sabai CORE:

C – Cardio Movement   _____

O – Optimum Hydration   _____

R – Rest and Recovery   _____

E – Eat Healthy   _____

WEEK 9 DAY 2: *Be Happy Now*

> *"I am the vine; you are the branches. The one who remains in me -- and I in him -- bears much fruit, because apart from me you can accomplish nothing. If you obey my commandments, you will remain in my love, just as I have obeyed my Father's commandments and remain in his love. I have told you these things so that my joy may be in you, and your joy may be complete. John 15:5,10-11 (NET)*

Related to "if / then" thinking is the idea that once we get healthy and lose the weight, we'll be happy.

Not true.

Your happiness isn't contingent on the scale. If you're not happy now, you won't be happy when you've lost the weight. As stated in John 15, you are fulfilled through Christ, through whom your joy is complete. Your happiness is most wrapped up in whether you consider yourself "successful" or not.

Are you happy?

During the past 9 weeks, you've done what many people won't! You've changed your eating habits. You've worked out consistently. You've gotten enough water and sleep to support your body. Be realistic in your self evaluation and give yourself credit.

You're a winner! You're the one that other's look to! You're the one that has set the example. If you don't see it yet, that's who you're becoming. Take pride in who you are, what you've come through, and what you're becoming. Let your joy be complete.

You're happy when you choose to be. When you choose to focus on what's great, in what you've accomplished, and the standards you've set.

Can you look yourself in the mirror and see a great person? Do you see the athlete developing in that body? Do you see a warrior who has come through tough times and continues to fight?

Choose to be proud of yourself. Be happy now!

WEEK 9 DAY 2: *Journal*

What are some wonderful things that you've accomplished in your life, in the past 8 weeks, and within the past day?

Life Accomplishment:

_____

Accomplishment during your Health With A Mission:

_____

Accomplishment during the past 24 hours:

_____

Happiness is a choice. The way you stand, what you choose to focus on, what you believe about yourself creates happiness. Choose to be happy now.

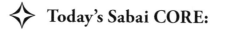 Today's Sabai CORE:

C – Cardio Movement   _____

O – Optimum Hydration   _____

R – Rest and Recovery   _____

E – Eat Healthy   _____

WEEK 9 DAY 3: *It's OK to Ask for Help*

Two blind men were sitting by the road. When they heard that Jesus was passing by, they shouted, "Have mercy on us, Lord, Son of David!" The crowd scolded them to get them to be quiet. But they shouted even more loudly, "Lord, have mercy on us, Son of David!" Jesus stopped, called them, and said, "What do you want me to do for you?" They said to him, "Lord, let our eyes be opened." Moved with compassion, Jesus touched their eyes. Immediately they received their sight and followed him. Matthew 20:30-34 (NET)

I can be a perfectionist at times. I also hate to ask for help. Doesn't that seem counterproductive to my goal of perfection?

As I look back on life, I realize that there are so many times that I've needed the help of others. I always need the help of Jesus. This journey to health is no different. Remember the beginning of my journey and the direction for this book came from crying out to God for help.

Whether you realize it or not, you're surrounded by resources. Ask for help! Pray that God gives you strength and wisdom. You will be blessed by resources if you ask. There are people who want you to succeed and do well. There are businesses dedicated to helping you become healthy. There are books with all wonderful information you can use to succeed in your journey.

If you knew all the answers, you probably wouldn't have picked up this book. That was a great step! Continue the momentum.

If you don't know what to do in the gym, ask a friend who works out successfully or hire a personal trainer! Join aerobics classes or get a video that you can work out with.

It's great to have a few workout friends. I have a friend I bicycle with occasionally, friends that like to go to the pool with me, and my wife loves to go for a run or walk with me. By enlisting the help of others, you are setting yourself up for success and encouragement.

When you ask for help, you're letting others know that they are important and you value their ideas and knowledge.

It helps to ask for help!

WEEK 9 DAY 3: *Journal*

What are some areas that you could use help in?

_____

_____

Who are some people or what are some resources that could give you the help that you need?

_____

_____

By finding the help and encouragement that you need, you're creating a path for success and accomplishment. Use the many resources at your fingertips to answer the questions, get the encouragement, and challenge you in your journey!

✦ Today's Sabai CORE:

C – Cardio Movement _____

O – Optimum Hydration _____

R – Rest and Recovery _____

E – Eat Healthy _____

WEEK 9 DAY 4: *Simplicity is Powerful*

For Christ did not send me to baptize, but to preach the gospel -- and not with clever speech, so that the cross of Christ would not become useless. For the message about the cross is foolishness to those who are perishing, but to us who are being saved it is the power of God. 1st Corinthians 1:17-18 (NET)

Part of the reason I don't count daily calories is that it makes my life more complicated. I used to design computer networks for large companies. I found that the more complicated I made a network, the more problematic it would be. The network administration team at the company couldn't maintain it properly, because it was too difficult to understand.

Your health plan is similar. If you make it complicated and hard to succeed, chances are that you'll fail. Keep your plan simple. The Sabai CORE is not complicated:

1. Exercise and movement daily.

2. Drink enough water daily. Your urine should remain light straw colored or clear.

3. A rest day each week and adequate sleep at night. You deserve it and your body needs it!

4. Eat healthy fresh foods, rich in vitamins and minerals. Stay away from processed foods that are "dead".

The reason this is powerful and works is the simplicity. You can make health more complicated if you want, but you don't have to.

Michael Jordan was one of the greatest basketball players ever. Even though he could make some incredible shots, most of his points came from doing the "basics" well.

As you continue your journey, practice the basics. Become an expert in consistently applying the Sabai CORE.

Simplicity is powerful!

Week 9 Day 4: *Journal*

What are simple things that you do create consistency in your Sabai CORE?

Cardio Movement:

_____

Optimum Hydration:

_____

Rest and Recovery:

_____

Eating Healthy:

_____

By keeping it simple, you avoid the traps of the "latest diet discovery" and other tricks that keep you unhealthy. Focus on simplicity through the Sabai CORE and your journey will continue and fitness will improve.

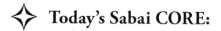 Today's Sabai CORE:

C – Cardio Movement   _____

O – Optimum Hydration   _____

R – Rest and Recovery   _____

E – Eat Healthy   _____

WEEK 9 DAY 5: *Why are you eating that?*

But a woman who had been suffering from a hemorrhage for twelve years came up behind him and touched the edge of his cloak. For she kept saying to herself, "If only I touch his cloak, I will be healed." But when Jesus turned and saw her he said, "Have courage, daughter! Your faith has made you well." And the woman was healed from that hour. Matthew 9:20-22 (NET)

In the evening, I'll sometimes have a small piece of dark chocolate. After a full day of workouts and healthy food, I enjoy my splurge as a way of celebrating a day lived well. That's ok.

Other times though, I have a strong desire for a gorge on chocolate, or chips, or fries, or something that's not healthy in quantity. That's not ok. When you feel compelled to eat, it's great to ask, "Why do I want this?" It's important to eat because of choice rather by compulsion.

If overeating is something that you've struggled with for years, reach out to Jesus and seek His healing touch. By asking in faith, you've made an important step that invites His help into your life. From that day when I asked for God's help, he has been with me as my comfort and strength.

When you want to eat, particularly when you are compelled to eat by a strong desire, ask yourself the question "Why am I hungry?" If it's not hunger, but a compulsion, reach out for God's help through prayer.

Here are some common reasons for the hunger urge:

- Boredom
- Past patterns
- To meet an emotional need
- To meet a sensory need
- Thirst for water
- Because it's time to refuel and eat

Each of the reasons above, except for the last one, can be met in a healthier way than eating. Meet the real need!

Week 9 Day 5: *Journal*

What are some times that you have felt compelled to eat when you're not hungry?

_____

_____

What is a healthy choice that would work for you instead?

_____

_____

Acknowledge yourself when you make a better choice. Many people go through life with their emotions and urges controlling their every action. You have chosen to acknowledge your emotions and urges and make healthy choices! That's a huge step forward!

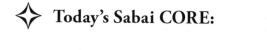 Today's Sabai CORE:

C – Cardio Movement   _____

O – Optimum Hydration   _____

R – Rest and Recovery   _____

E – Eat Healthy   _____

WEEK 9 DAY 6: *The Program or the Health?*

When they came to Mysia, they attempted to go into Bithynia, but the Spirit of Jesus did not allow them to do this, so they passed through Mysia and went down to Troas. A vision appeared to Paul during the night: A Macedonian man was standing there urging him, "Come over to Macedonia and help us!" After Paul saw the vision, we attempted immediately to go over to Macedonia, concluding that God had called us to proclaim the good news to them. Acts 16:7-10 (NET)

Continue asking the question, "What's the healthy choice?" Making the healthy choice sometimes means adjusting our plans. Eating and exercise plans should never take priority over your health. They serve you by building into your fitness. If they ever start detracting from your health, then you need to make changes.

In our verses today, Paul had been traveling to proclaim the good news but had been hitting walls. They planned to go to Bithynia but the Spirit blocked them. In seeking God's best, a vision came to Paul and he followed it. He changed his good plans to achieve the highest goal.

One day, during a strong run, I injured my knee. Rather than "pushing through the pain", I adjusted my plan and substituted swimming until the knee had healed. I changed good plans to achieve a higher goal.

Part of being unhealthy is being out of touch with your body and its needs. Practice "listening" to your body, evaluate what you're hearing, and make healthy choices to meet the needs.

The important principles are to hear your body and make a wise decision that supports building health.

Let's say your body is screaming for a piece of chocolate pound cake. First acknowledge the urge. Then consider what that means. Did you have a healthy snack between meals or did you go too long without eating? Are you getting enough calories in your eating plan, or have you been denying yourself in an effort to speed up the process? Has it been too long since your last splurge?

Evaluate the signals your body sends and make wise decisions that support health!

WEEK 9 DAY 6: *Journal*

Is there an aspect of your journey which is currently out of balance? Are you pushing too hard in one area or ignoring part of the Sabai CORE?

_____

_____

_____

If there are areas of imbalance, what are some changes you'll make, starting now?

_____

_____

_____

By adjusting when you've pushed too hard in one area, you are learning to listen to your body and give it the healthy solutions it craves!

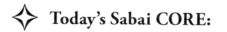 **Today's Sabai CORE:**

C – Cardio Movement   _____

O – Optimum Hydration   _____

R – Rest and Recovery   _____

E – Eat Healthy   _____

WEEK 9 DAY 7: *Focus, Choices, and Outcome*

> *So he said, "Come." Peter got out of the boat, walked on the water, and came toward Jesus. But when he saw the strong wind he became afraid. And starting to sink, he cried out, "Lord, save me!" Immediately Jesus reached out his hand and caught him, saying to him, "You of little faith, why did you doubt?" When they went up into the boat, the wind ceased. Then those who were in the boat worshiped him, saying, "Truly you are the Son of God." Matthew 14:29-33 (NET)*

Once I took a Skip Barber Racing School and I remember well a piece of advice they gave. They said to always focus your eyes on where you want to go. If you lose control and fix your focus onto a tree, you'll hit it! If you focus on the road, you'd regain control. Isn't that true in life? Do you know someone who is always focused on what's wrong in life? They get a horrible result from a horrible focus. Consider today's verses. When Peter was focused on Jesus, he was walking on water! When he focused on the waves, he began to sink.

I often ask my kids "What was great about today?" That's a wonderful question because it forces you to take a look at what's great in life.

We all have things to be thankful for. We also have struggles and challenges that we could resent. The difference is what you choose to focus on.

By suggesting that you focus on what is great, I am not advocating ignoring problems or issues. It is unhealthy to ignore problems or pretend they don't exist. It is also unhealthy to give them primary focus and define yourself by those issues. So often our focus tends to be on what we've done wrong and where we've missed the mark. It's not healthy to be focused on where you've been, rather than where you're going.

There's a saying that it's hard to move forward while focused on the rear view mirror. That's true in your life and journey toward health. Whether you've made poor choices in the past is not relevant to your destination! Isn't that an amazing statement?

Your focus will determine your choices. Your choices will determine your outcome. By keeping your focus on what's great in life and where you want to go, you'll "steer" your life in that direction!

WEEK 9 DAY 7: *Journal*

Are there areas in your life where your focus is taking you down an unhealthy path? If so, what?

_____

_____

_____

What can you re-focus on that will take you where you want to go and give you great results?

_____

_____

_____

By resetting your focus on where you want to go and the results that you want to achieve, you set yourself up for success and accomplishment! Keep your eyes on what's great in life and empowers you.

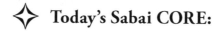 **Today's Sabai CORE:**

C – Cardio Movement   _____

O – Optimum Hydration   _____

R – Rest and Recovery   _____

E – Eat Healthy   _____

WEEK 10 DAY 1: *Turn Negatives, Positive*

Now obey the LORD and worship him with integrity and loyalty. Put aside the gods your ancestors worshiped beyond the Euphrates and in Egypt and worship the LORD. If you have no desire to worship the LORD, choose today whom you will worship, whether it be the gods whom your ancestors worshiped beyond the Euphrates, or the gods of the Amorites in whose land you are living. But I and my family will worship the LORD!" The people responded, "Far be it from us to abandon the LORD so we can worship other gods! For the LORD our God took us and our fathers out of slavery in the land of Egypt and performed these awesome miracles before our very eyes. He continually protected us as we traveled and when we passed through nations. Joshua 24:14-17 (NET)

In life, tough times will happen. We all have setbacks along the way. Learn how to use the negative experiences as a catalyst to create something positive in your life.

My Mom struggled with her weight throughout her life. Recently, I learned that a month before she died from cancer she went to the doctor as required by her chemotherapy treatments. They weighed her and the scale showed 175 pounds. "Finally", she whispered in a weak voice, "I've hit my goal weight."

How sad that it took the ravages of cancer and aggressive chemotherapy treatments for my Mom to hit her "goal weight". She died a month later.

The choice is the lesson I will take from the experience. I could remain in sadness and how "unfair" it was that she never got to enjoy a healthy weight or I can decide that I will reach a healthy weight with time to enjoy that health with my family and friends.

Use the tough times in life to learn important lessons that carry your toward your goals. I'm always inspired by those who can take incredibly challenging situations and circumstances and rise above with an empowering lesson taken from the experience.

Joshua knew God's people had gone through tough times. He also knew that God had delivered them and his family.

Use tough times to gain strength! You'll gain valuable lessons and inspire others in the process.

Turn the negatives, positive.

Week 10 Day 1: *Journal*

When was a tough time that gave you valuable lessons for life?

_____

_____

_____

What is a negative lesson that you have learned from a past experience that you could rework into the positive?

_____

_____

_____

No matter how difficult your past or present circumstances, they can be used for the good of yourself and others. Use the tough times as fuel to help those around you, including yourself.

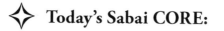 Today's Sabai CORE:

C – Cardio Movement _____

O – Optimum Hydration _____

R – Rest and Recovery _____

E – Eat Healthy _____

Week 10 Day 2: *Love Yourself Now*

> *"Teacher, which commandment in the law is the greatest?" Jesus said to him, " 'Love the Lord your God with all your heart, with all your soul, and with all your mind.' This is the first and greatest commandment. The second is like it: 'Love your neighbor as yourself.' All the law and the prophets depend on these two commandments." Matthew 22:36-40 (NET)*

We often notice in these verses the command to love God or love our neighbor but the third part is overlooked. We're to love our neighbor *as we love ourselves.*

Without loving ourselves, we cannot love others well. Many people make loving themselves a prize to be given after reaching the "goal". You don't have to wait!

Choose to love yourself now. Whether you are at your goal weight range or you have 100 pounds to lose, you are special, loved and designed by God, and incredibly valuable. There is amazing opportunity ahead in your life and God has a plan for your future.

Why is loving yourself important? It's actually critical to gaining health. Disliking self is destructive. We have all seen stories in the news of people who use their dislike of themselves as reasoning to destroy others.

When you love yourself and give grace when mistakes are made, you've created a clear path for health to develop in your life. You've also set a great example for others who look to you for leadership, like your children, spouse, and coworkers.

When you fully realize that God designed you, loves you and has a plan for your future, you are compelled to love yourself. If you didn't, you would be dishonoring God's design.

Give yourself the same care and respect that you would give a friend that you admire and love. Love yourself now!

Week 10 Day 2: *Journal*

Do you love yourself as much as you love others?

_____

_____

_____

What are actions you can take which express love to yourself in a healthy way?

_____

_____

_____

It's impossible to be truly healthy if there is not love of self. Being healthy means caring for and loving self in a balanced way. Love yourself and you'll gain momentum in your journey.

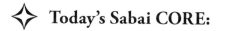 Today's Sabai CORE:

C – Cardio Movement   _____

O – Optimum Hydration   _____

R – Rest and Recovery   _____

E – Eat Healthy   _____

WEEK 10 DAY 3: *Stretch*

I rejoice in the lifestyle prescribed by your rules as if they were riches of all kinds. I will meditate on your precepts and focus on your behavior. Psalms 119:14-15 (NET)

After years of lethargy and getting into couch potato form, my body just wasn't very flexible. For type "A" personalities that want to get on with the workout, it seems difficult to justify the time to stretch. Wouldn't that time be better spent lifting some weights or running a mile?

The reality is no. Stretching and balance are closely linked. By becoming more flexible, you are also giving your body options of movement to choose from. Stretching will give you a wider range of motion and help protect your muscles and joints from damage.

Use your time stretching to slow down, relax, and focus on what's great in your life. Think of your progress made, what your healthy body will look like within its goal weight range, or any other aspect of life that is positive and uplifting. Meditate on God's truth, as described in today's Psalm.

Stretching is a great time to reflect and care for you. It's a great time for prayer and listening to God's response.

Here's how to start:

- Wear clothing that allows a full range of motion
- Start with fluid movements that fall within your typical range of motion.
- Go ahead and do your regular exercise.
- Following the exercise, do some "static" stretches which take your body just a little further than it was able to go before your exercise.

Stretching will give you flexibility! It also gives you time to slow down and seek God.

Week 10 Day 3: *Journal*

How would you rate your flexibility today, on a scale of one to ten?

1 _____ 10

Stretching will lead to increased flexibility over time. It can be done as part of a workout routine, as in yoga, or before and after a workout. How do you plan to implement stretching into your daily routine?

_____

_____

_____

As you become more flexible, you receive multiple benefits. You have muscles engaging to keep you balanced. You are less prone to injury and falls. You are also able to easily tie your shoes! I have loved the flexibility that gaining health has given!

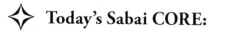 **Today's Sabai CORE:**

C – Cardio Movement _____

O – Optimum Hydration _____

R – Rest and Recovery _____

E – Eat Healthy _____

Week 10 Day 4: *Exercise Balance!*

A wise warrior is strong, and a man of knowledge makes his strength stronger; for with guidance you wage your war, and with numerous advisers there is victory. Proverbs 25:5-6 (NET)

Balance is so important and elusive; we should spend a second day focused on it. While it's a rare moment we're ever completely in balance, balance is the place that you want to constantly move toward.

When you were unhealthy, you were out of balance physically. As you are working on your Sabai CORE daily, you are now working toward a healthy balance.

The interesting thing about balance is that it is difficult to maintain. It requires an ongoing effort and focus.

This begs the following question, "Why we should strive for something that requires ongoing effort and focus?"

When we're not striving for balance, it is natural to become grossly unbalanced. Think of it like a number line from -10 to 0 to +10. If 0 is balanced and both the other extremes are out of balance, our natural inclination is to drift toward one extreme or the other.

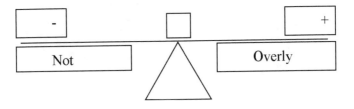

I've had times when I've pushed too hard in my training and moved into the + side, and times when I've not been motivated and moved into the – side.

Strive for balance, it will serve you well.

Week 10 Day 4: *Journal*

What are some areas of your life where you feel that you are in balance?

_____

_____

_____

What are some areas of your life where you are currently out of balance?

_____

_____

_____

What actions can you take to bring those areas into balance?

_____

_____

_____

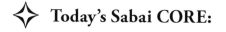 **Today's Sabai CORE:**

C – Cardio Movement   _____

O – Optimum Hydration   _____

R – Rest and Recovery   _____

E – Eat Healthy   _____

WEEK 10 DAY 5: *Away from/toward*

Not only this, but we also rejoice in sufferings, knowing that suffering produces endurance, and endurance, character, and character, hope. And hope does not disappoint, because the love of God has been poured out in our hearts through the Holy Spirit who was given to us. Romans 5:3-5

People are motivated by avoiding pain or gaining pleasure. These are two basic drives that affect us all but they work in very different ways.

Avoiding pain / away from - We will do more to avoid pain in the short term. Over time, we will either successfully move away from the pain or become desensitized to the pain and learn to accept it.

Gaining Pleasure / Moving Toward – Moving toward something that gives pleasure will work much more effectively as a long term motivation. One of the reasons that a moving toward goal works better in the long term is that it helps create patterns of success.

You may remember from my introduction at the beginning of this book, my initial motivation was to avoid pain. I was sick of "being fat". While that was very strong motivation for the first week or two, I was already tired of the effort by the end of the first month.

That is when I was able to make the shift toward gaining health. As a motivation, gaining health is far more effective goal because it is something that you gain pleasure from and move toward.

If your motivation is to avoid being seen as fat, having your husband leave you, embarrassing your children, or any other pain then your efforts will be short lived. In our verse today, even the suffering is focused on the hope. The challenges are a path toward achieving the goal.

Consider how you can shift this motivation toward health. You could be driven to look great for your spouse, healthy and able to play with your kids and setting a great example for family and friends. These are all such positive goals to move toward.

What is it you're moving toward? Rather than moving away from the negatives, move toward the positive result you design. Gain health!

WEEK 10 DAY 5: *Journal*

What is your primary motivation for working through this book?

_____

Is that motivation something you're moving away from or toward? For example, "so I won't be fat" or "I won't be embarrassed in a swimsuit" are both "away from" goals. "So I'll be strong and healthy" or "I'll look incredibly fit in a swimsuit" are both positive moving toward goals.

_____

Write a positive moving toward goal for your journey.

_____

_____

_____

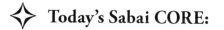 **Today's Sabai CORE:**

C – Cardio Movement   _____

O – Optimum Hydration   _____

R – Rest and Recovery   _____

E – Eat Healthy   _____

Week 10 Day 6: *Serenity*

The LORD is my shepherd, I lack nothing. He takes me to lush pastures, he leads me to refreshing water. He restores my strength. He leads me down the right paths for the sake of his reputation. Even when I must walk through the darkest valley, I fear no danger, for you are with me; your rod and your staff reassure me. You prepare a feast before me in plain sight of my enemies. You refresh my head with oil; my cup is completely full. Surely your goodness and faithfulness will pursue me all my days, and I will live in the LORD's house for the rest of my life. Psalm 23 (NET)

Serenity is a one of those things that is hard to describe but easy to identify. These are some words that are related: peaceful, loving, confident, flexible, perceptive and balanced. Sounds pretty good doesn't it?

Gaining health physically will bring you closer to a sense of serenity but physical health alone cannot achieve it. True serenity comes from having health physically, mentally, and spiritually. Part of this process is identifying ways to gain health in each of these areas.

If you're physically fit but mentally a mess, you will not have a good quality of life. If you are physically health but lack a spiritual dimension, you're missing the whole point!

Imagine you've worked hard and your body reflects the effort. As you return from the gym, you enter a messy house and get in a fight with your spouse. You're mad at God because you've prayed for change and nothing is better. That's not serenity.

Imagine instead that you've worked hard and your body reflects the effort. You come home from the gym to a house that reflects your interests and love. Pictures on the wall show places you've been and people you love. Your spouse has had a tough day and you know that sitting down and hearing her struggles will be great for her and bring you closer. After dinner, and as the evening ends, you feel blessed that you have this spouse, this home, and this life. You thank God for His blessings and direction in life.

Serenity comes from focus and time spent on what's important in life. What are the challenges that you need to face to gain serenity?

WEEK 10 DAY 6: *Journal*

How would you rate your serenity level today, on a scale of one to ten?

1 _____ 10

What are some actions you can take that will increase your sense of serenity and peace?

_____

_____

_____

Gaining serenity may come from changes internally but often come from helping those around you. Note in the example on the prior page that by helping a spouse after a tough day, both of you have an increased sense of peace.

✦ Today's Sabai CORE:

C – Cardio Movement _____

O – Optimum Hydration _____

R – Rest and Recovery _____

E – Eat Healthy _____

Week 10 Day 7: *Cracked Heels*

Now a man was there who had been disabled for thirty-eight years. When Jesus saw him lying there and when he realized that the man had been disabled a long time already, he said to him, "Do you want to become well?" The sick man answered him, "Sir, I have no one to put me into the pool when the water is stirred up. While I am trying to get into the water, someone else goes down there before me." Jesus said to him, "Stand up! Pick up your mat and walk." Immediately the man was healed, and he picked up his mat and started walking. (Now that day was a Sabbath.) John 5:5-9 (NET)

I'm sure that some of you did a double take when you saw the title of this lesson. What do I mean "Cracked Heels"?

Let me explain it this way…

Over the years, the skin on my feet grew so thick and calloused that cracks began to develop in the thick skin. As the skin grew drier, cracks would deepen to the point where my heels would be in severe pain when I walked. My feet hurt for over a decade from these cracks.

I had developed a sense of learned helplessness about my feet. The truth is that cracked heels are a common problem with several remedies that keep them from becoming a severe problem. I just wasn't implementing the solutions.

What are the "Cracked Feet" in your life? What are the lingering problems and issues that you've resigned yourself to? In today's scripture, the man had been disabled for thirty-eight years! Note that he didn't even ask Jesus for healing, just for help to the water. Are you seeking help for your lingering issues?

As we're gaining health, it's important to see the areas in our life that we've allowed to be perpetually unhealthy. Perhaps you have a relationship that needs healing and forgiveness. Perhaps you've let credit card debt become an ongoing burden. Perhaps you have a simple problem like cracked heels.

Work on gaining health involves all aspects of your life, including physical, financial, spiritual, and relationships.

Today I give my heels regular care and they are a reminder that I'm gaining health in many ways!

Week 10 Day 7: *Journal*

What are some issues other than weight that you can begin addressing? What are some of the steps you can take to move toward a solution?

Issue   Step toward solution

_____   _____

_____   _____

_____   _____

Sometimes you'll need to find books or other resources to work toward the solutions to your "cracked feet". Find resources that focus on addressing the root issues in a healthy manner.

When the disabled man got help from Jesus, he immediately got up and started walking. In your issue, what will you be able to do once healing is underway?

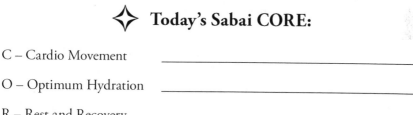

✦ Today's Sabai CORE:

C – Cardio Movement   _____

O – Optimum Hydration   _____

R – Rest and Recovery   _____

E – Eat Healthy   _____

WEEK 11 DAY 1: *Why – Part one...*

Therefore I exhort you, brothers and sisters, by the mercies of God, to present your bodies as a sacrifice -- alive, holy, and pleasing to God -- which is your reasonable service. Romans 12:1 (NET)

What's your why?

Why is it crucial that you gain health? Why are you dedicated to this journey? Why will you remain faithful to your health despite any setbacks?

These questions are important because your "why" is what keeps you in the game when things are rough. If your answer is external like "so my husband will think I look sexy" or "so others won't think I'm fat", consider finding a different answer.

Your "why" is as personal as your body is. Your "why" needs to become as long term and personal as this journey is.

My initial 'why' was "because I'm sick of being fat". The answer has become "because this body is a gift that I treasure and enjoy". What a difference the answer makes!

As the answer has shifted, so has my body perception. From disgusted to appreciative is a pretty wide range! It's a lot more fun to treasure and enjoy your body and its capabilities. The outcome of a healthy "why" is a healthy body that supports a great life.

Often we need to make decisions with our head before they become part of our heart. Consider your "why" and what one would be that will support you long term. Your "why" is your drive and motivation that helps keep you grounded when the day is tough.

What is your "why"?

Week 11 Day 1: *Journal*

What is your "why" that has driven you through to week 11 in this book?

_____

_____

_____

Is the "why" powerful and empowering? _____ Is it personal or focused on others?_____

Write your "why" in powerful, positive, and powerful language.

_____

_____

_____

By having a why that is personal and positive, you develop an internal drive that is not dependent on external circumstances.

✦ Today's Sabai CORE:

C – Cardio Movement   _____

O – Optimum Hydration   _____

R – Rest and Recovery   _____

E – Eat Healthy   _____

WEEK 11 DAY 2: *Why – Part Two*

Do not be conformed to this present world, but be transformed by the renewing of your mind, so that you may test and approve what is the will of God -- what is good and well-pleasing and perfect. Romans 12:2 (NET)

Sometimes there is can be a subconscious "why" that has helped create the weight issue.

Growing up in a family with four kids meant that if I didn't eat quickly, I couldn't get seconds. They'd be all gone! While this shouldn't have had a huge effect on my life 35 years later, it did. I found myself in negative eating patterns established when I was young.

The challenge is that I'm no longer sitting at a dinner table with my young brothers and sister. I sit at my own family table and don't really need to worry about whether seconds are available.

I've heard people tell stories of getting comfort from food after a traumatic experience in childhood. Food may have been used by a Mom or aunt to show love in a time of need. Guilt may have been used when plates weren't cleaned off.

Do any of these sound familiar? Perhaps you have a "why-part two" that has guided your relationship with food over the years.

By identifying these driving forces behind your eating, you can address the lies that you still believe and replace those lies with the truth.

The truth is that you can make your own choices. The truth is that any past time of scarcity is over. The truth is that love can be shown in a multitude of ways, not just food.

What is your "Why- part two"?

WEEK 11 DAY 2: *Journal*

Is there a why established that isn't based on logic, but on your past?_____ If so, identify your "why-part two".

_____

_____

_____

What is the lie that why is based on? For example, mine was that "food is scarce and you better get it now!" Food was no longer scarce and I didn't need to horde.

_____

What is the truth that is healthy and helps you create a vibrant life? For example, mine is that "food is so abundant; I should only choose what I really want."

_____

_____

_____

✦ Today's Sabai CORE:

C – Cardio Movement   _____

O – Optimum Hydration   _____

R – Rest and Recovery   _____

E – Eat Healthy   _____

Week 11 Day 3: *Success Creates Success*

This brings you great joy, although you may have to suffer for a short time in various trials. Such trials show the proven character of your faith, which is much more valuable than gold -- gold that is tested by fire, even though it is passing away -- and will bring praise and glory and honor when Jesus Christ is revealed. You have not seen him, but you love him. You do not see him now but you believe in him, and so you rejoice with an indescribable and glorious joy, because you are attaining the goal of your faith -- the salvation of your souls. 1ˢᵗ Peter 1:6-9 (NET)

Positive momentum is a situation where success creates success. When you begin anything, there is an enormous effort needed to get started. At first you may fail a time or two but then, once you begin succeeding it becomes easier to succeed again. Over time, what seemed difficult or even insurmountable becomes easy and natural to accomplish.

Imagine a violinist. In the beginning, it is difficult to hit the right notes. Later timing must be mastered. Eventually, a piece by Mozart that would have been impossible becomes second nature.

Living healthy has the same learning curve. In the beginning weeks and months of developing a healthy lifestyle it may seem awkward. It takes such an effort to get to the gym or pull out the workout video. Over time, the workouts that were impossible become too easy and you need a bigger challenge.

As you continue to gain health, you will learn patterns that work for you. By keeping a set of workout clothes in the car, you are always ready to stop at the gym. By waking 30 minutes earlier, you have the time for a morning workout. By connecting with your gym buddies, the time there is fun. These are all "successes" and by continuing habits that work for you, you are creating a framework for continued success.

What was initially awkward will eventually be second nature. Living a healthy lifestyle is becoming a natural pattern, an extension of who you are.

Success creates success.

Week 11 Day 3: *Journal*

What are some examples of positive momentum in your life?

_____

_____

_____

_____

_____

What are some actions you can take to increase your positive momentum in gaining health?

_____

_____

_____

_____

By "feeding the momentum" that you've developed, you make it easier to accomplish your goals. Identify the patterns and choices that help you succeed!

✦ Today's Sabai CORE:

C – Cardio Movement　　_____

O – Optimum Hydration　_____

R – Rest and Recovery　　_____

E – Eat Healthy　　　　　_____

Week 11 Day 4: *Involving Others*

"Which one of you, if he has a hundred sheep and loses one of them, would not leave the ninety-nine in the open pasture and go look for the one that is lost until he finds it? Then when he has found it, he places it on his shoulders, rejoicing. Returning home, he calls together his friends and neighbors, telling them, 'Rejoice with me, because I have found my sheep that was lost.'
Luke 15:4-6 (NET)

As you are gaining health and your waist is shrinking, chances are you'll have to go shopping for some new clothes. Don't go alone!

You want this journey to be one that the important people in your life can celebrate with you. Whether they're gaining health with you or just watching from the sidelines, involve them in the celebrations.

Healthy romantic relationship require love and caring for each other without preconditions. What if your spouse or sweetheart isn't currently on the same journey to health that you've begun? That's ok! This journey isn't about fixing anyone else or even pointing out where they should improve. If you focus on your health, others will want to follow but first they're going test you.

- Will you still love them if they don't make changes as well?
- Are they more important than your exercise and food plan?
- Are you going to finish what you started?
- Can you keep this up over time?
- Are you going to get healthy in all areas, including temper, relationships, and finances?

These are reasonable questions for your loved ones to be asking. Ensure that you don't become an obstacle to others by trying to force them down the road you're on. Focus on gaining health for yourself and being healthy in your relationships.

By loving others as you love yourself you'll set a precedent that others can follow.

WEEK 11 DAY 4: *Journal*

Who are the people that you most want to share this journey with?

_____

_____

_____

_____

What are some ways that you can share your changes in a way that encourages them as well?

_____

_____

_____

_____

By involving those you love, you get to develop a support circle around you. When they see that your fitness doesn't mean thinking less of them, they can begin supporting and loving your changes!

✦ Today's Sabai CORE:

C – Cardio Movement _____

O – Optimum Hydration _____

R – Rest and Recovery _____

E – Eat Healthy _____

Week 11 Day 5: *Mini goals you control*

> *So Samuel led Israel all the days of his life. Year after year he used to travel the circuit of Bethel, Gilgal, and Mizpah; he used to judge Israel in all of these places. Then he would return to Ramah, because his home was there. He also judged Israel there and built an altar to the Lord there. 1ˢᵗ Samuel 7:15-17 (NET)*

What is the date what you will first enter your healthy weight range? Unless you've entered that weight range already, it's almost impossible to tell. It's great to set goals and much better to assign a date to accomplish that goal. When you have a large and long-term goal established, how do you accomplish it? Mini-goals that take you that direction!

That is really what we're doing in this book and through your process of "gaining health". We've committed to a significant task and then developed mini goals that take you that direction. Drinking adequate water is a simple and measurable mini goal that takes you in the right direction. Eating lots of fresh veggies and fruit is a mini goal that can be measured and easily achieved. The same goes for exercise and rest. Doing each day's lesson and journal is a mini goal which breaks down into weeks and months.

Whether you have a goal of running a 5k or competing in an Ironman, that goal can be achieved by focusing on mini goals that are easily achievable, take you toward the goal, and can be measured to assure that they've been achieved. What may seem like a daunting task is achievable as a series of mini goals.

In today's verses, Samuel had a number of tasks that he established in his life that allowed him to rule effectively and be consistent in worshipping his God. He moved from responsibility to responsibility, or you might say, goal to goal.

The coolrunning.com website developed a program called "Couch to 5k", which is a training program designed to take someone from couch potato to a 5k runner in 8 weeks. This program is a series of mini goals that create the desired outcome.

Consider what your goals are in health, family, work and any other area you are developing. Design the mini goals that will take you toward your outcome. Focus on mini goals that you control!

Week 11 Day 5: *Journal*

What is a big goal that you could break into mini goals?

_____

What are some mini goals that are easily achievable that you can set that will move you toward your big goal?

1. _____

2. _____

3. _____

By setting mini goals that are challenging yet achievable within a short time frame, you are guaranteeing momentum in your major goals!

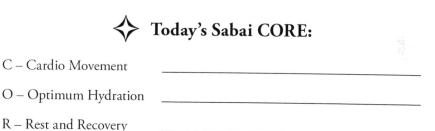 **Today's Sabai CORE:**

C – Cardio Movement _____

O – Optimum Hydration _____

R – Rest and Recovery _____

E – Eat Healthy _____

WEEK 11 DAY 6: *Identity times two*

So then, if anyone is in Christ, he is a new creation; what is old has passed away -- look, what is new has come! 2ⁿᵈ Corinthians 5:17 (NET)

In an earlier chapter we talked about identity and the shift needed for long term change.

There's more than one identity that will need to change and sometimes it's this other one that's more problematic. It's the identity that your friends, family, and co-workers have of you.

While we know that our friends and family care for us, that doesn't always mean that they are excited about us becoming healthy. Why? Because many times that shakes their identity and puts them in a very uncomfortable place.

This morning my wife, Cindy, and I were running and she said that she had always seen herself as skinnier than me (and rightfully so!). As the weight started dropping off my frame, she realized that unless she made changes that identity wouldn't stand.

What if Cindy hadn't been willing to make those changes? There could have been an unspoken unease between us as my weight dropped.

Are there others in your life whose self identity is being shaken by your weight loss? If so, take the time to let them know you love them. Perhaps they don't need to hear about the last five pounds that came off.

I've really enjoyed being in online communities like ours at www.healthwithamission.com or www.sparkpeople.com where I'm surrounded by others making the same types of changes in their lives.

By changing your identity, others re-evaluate theirs.

WEEK 11 DAY 6: *Journal*

What are three words that you think others would use to describe you?

1. _____ 2. _____ 3. _____

Ask someone who cares about you to give you three words that they would use to describe you.

1. _____ 2. _____ 3. _____

Are there shifts in your identity that will happen as you continue in your journey? What are new words you want people to be using in a year?

1. _____ 2. _____ 3. _____

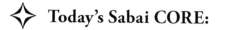 Today's Sabai CORE:

C – Cardio Movement   _____

O – Optimum Hydration   _____

R – Rest and Recovery   _____

E – Eat Healthy   _____

WEEK 11 DAY 7: *Never Give up!*

"I am determined, O God! I am determined! I will sing and praise you!" Psalms 57:7 (NET)

Imagine that one day coming home from work late, you fall asleep on the couch, waking the next morning. As you wake, you realize that you forgot to brush your teeth before you went to sleep. Disgusted with yourself for your lack of control and discipline, you realize that you are a failure at oral hygiene. You throw away your toothbrush and decide it's just too hard to try to succeed in the face of such failure.

Crazy scenario, isn't it? Isn't that what SO many people do with their plans to get fit? After a tough day or weekend, they "toss in the towel" and label themselves a failure at the process.

You haven't failed unless you quit! Fitness isn't a race but a lifelong event. As long as you're striving, changing, learning, and choosing this path, you're succeeding.

You have already done what many people will not. You have stayed with this process for at least eleven weeks, as you're on this lesson! You have already established a discipline that will serve you well. I may have given you some tools but you are the one who has picked them up and used them.

The story of Joni Erickson Tada is a great example of persistence through the trials. After an accident left her paralyzed, she eventually learned to paint and write with a pen in her mouth and has blessed countless lives with her testimony.

In the darkest days of World War II, Winston Churchill stated "Never give in. Never give in. Never, never, never, never--in nothing, great or small, large or petty--never give in, except to convictions of honor and good sense."

You are on the right path. You have shown fortitude and strength. You have shown persistence and courage.

Never give up!

WEEK 11 DAY 7: *Journal*

List the character traits that have brought you this far on the journey: *Example:*
determination, courage.

_____

_____

_____

Describe how these character traits will keep you on the path when the times
are tough? *Example: my determination will bring me through even when I don't*
"feel like it".

_____

_____

_____

Acknowledging the strengths that you've developed and use those strengths
to succeed. You have character traits that have brought you this far and those
same strengths will lead you to continued success!

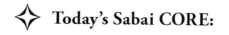 **Today's Sabai CORE:**

C – Cardio Movement _____

O – Optimum Hydration _____

R – Rest and Recovery _____

E – Eat Healthy _____

WEEK 12 DAY 1: *The Lost Weekend*

> *But I say, live by the Spirit and you will not carry out the desires of the flesh. For the flesh has desires that are opposed to the Spirit, and the Spirit has desires that are opposed to the flesh, for these are in opposition to each other, so that you cannot do what you want. But if you are led by the Spirit, you are not under the law. Galatians 5:16-18 (NET)*

In 1945 there was a great film, which won an Oscar, called "The Lost Weekend" that chronicled a weekend binge of an alcoholic.

One weekend, well into my journey I had a "lost weekend" of my own. It wasn't with alcohol but instead with food. On top of eating whatever I wanted, I didn't exercise either! For some reason, I just ate to my heart's content and watched TV.

I'd recently finished a vacation time where I had done great. I'd maintained my weight loss and even lost a little more during the vacation. I was getting back in the rhythm of daily workouts. By the end of my "lost weekend", the losses of the past week and a half were erased on the scale.

Why did I do this? I think it had something to do with choice. I decided that I could, so I would. It may not be the brightest rationale but it was my reasoning. A couple of things helped keep it from becoming a lost week or month.

- Continuing to weigh myself.
- Realizing that I felt worse, not better.

By acknowledging the "lost weekend" and the fitness lost, I was able to choose health. Gaining health is an ongoing choice that we make for ourselves. Over the following weeks with renewed workouts and healthy eating, I was right back on track.

This journey isn't about any day or weekend but about the long run.

Week 12 Day 1: *Journal*

What are some ways that you can recover from a lost day or weekend? What are some actions you'll take as soon as you realize that you're off track?

1. _____

2. _____

3. _____

By thinking ahead and planning your response when you get off track, you make the recovery from those times fast and empowering. We all have down times and challenges in life, how we recover and make it through those times is where the difference lies.

✦ Today's Sabai CORE:

C – Cardio Movement _____

O – Optimum Hydration _____

R – Rest and Recovery _____

E – Eat Healthy _____

WEEK 12 DAY 2: *Do a Double!*

But those who wait for the Lord's help find renewed strength;
they rise up as if they had eagles' wings, they run without growing
weary, they walk without getting tired. Isaiah 40:31(NET)

Sometimes we get silly stuff stuck in our head. Remember a couple of months ago; exercising an hour in a day was a stretch! Don't let those stretches become an upper limit. There's nothing magical about an hour but it's a reasonable amount of time to focus on caring for your health each day.

What if it was an hour and a half? You'd be surprised to see the speed at which change will happen. By doing a "double", or adding in a second workout, you'll increase the speed at which you're defining your body.

Triathletes call back-to-back double workouts "bricks". Because of the nature of that sport, doing different workouts in the same day is par for the course. It trains your muscles to "expect the unexpected" and prepare for being needed. It also increased your calorie burn rate for an extended period over the day.

You can do a double occasionally, to mix things up, or you can do a double every day! In May 2008, after losing over 100 pounds, I had hit a plateau. By adding in a 25 minute aerobic video to my daily workouts, the pounds started dropping off again.

My regular workouts have consisted of biking or running, elliptical trainer and weights, with occasional swims. Adding on this 25 minute video workout at a different time of the day increased variety in the workouts, increased my metabolism, and increased the speed of the changes being made!

See what you think. Come on, do a double!

Week 12 Day 2: *Journal*

During the coming week, consider doing a double! If you choose to accept this assignment, write down the day and workout, and second workout:

Date: _____

Workout: _____

Workout 2: _____

Doubles will help you pick up the pace and can help get you off a frustrating plateau. You can call it a "brick" and get quizzical looks from your workout buddies.

✦ Today's Sabai CORE:

C – Cardio Movement   _____

O – Optimum Hydration   _____

R – Rest and Recovery   _____

E – Eat Healthy   _____

Week 12 Day 3: *Be Playful*

"Now David, wearing a linen ephod, was dancing with all his strength before the Lord. David and all Israel were bringing up the ark of the Lord, shouting and blowing trumpets." I Samuel 6:14-15 (NET)

When is the last time you were playful? I'm hoping that you can think of an example in the past week! If you can't, then you should consider doing something fun...

Sitting at home in front of the TV is not an activity. It's a non-activity. Most of the time, it just doesn't accomplish much. Much of the programming is like junk food for the brain. It fills your time and doesn't leave you satisfied.

Here are some of the playful things I've done since beginning of this journey.

- Gone running and enjoyed it like a kid.
- Ridden my bike and gone exploring.
- Taken a kayak out on the ocean.
- Done geocaching with the family.
- Gone elephant riding.
- Ride my motorcycle into the countryside.
- Gone bowling with the kids.
- Done a "ropes course" 25 meters high.
- Gone swimming many times.
- Walks on the beach.
- Gone for picnics and outings with the family.
- Run a triathlon with friends.
- Had friends over for dinners.

We are so blessed to have health and our life in front of us. Acknowledge the gift and enjoy it. Did you ever roll down a hill of grass when you were a kid? Roll around in life laughing with your friends! Embrace the gift you've been given.

Be playful!

WEEK 12 DAY 3: *Journal*

List some playful things that you've done in your life:

_____

_____

_____

Choose one playful thing that you choose to do this coming week:

_____

If you give this a half-hearted effort, you'll get a half-hearted result. When you choose to do something, do it with your full effort. Have fun and play "full out"!

The more playful you are, the more joyous the journey.

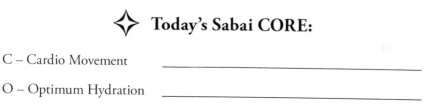 Today's Sabai CORE:

C – Cardio Movement   _____

O – Optimum Hydration   _____

R – Rest and Recovery   _____

E – Eat Healthy   _____

Week 12 Day 4: *Posture*

Therefore, since we are surrounded by such a great cloud of witnesses, we must get rid of every weight and the sin that clings so closely, and run with endurance the race set out for us, keeping our eyes fixed on Jesus, the pioneer and perfecter of our faith. For the joy set out for him he endured the cross, disregarding its shame, and has taken his seat at the right hand of the throne of God. Hebrews 12:1-2 (NET)

Imagine a strong and athletic person walking toward you. Is her head up or down? Is she standing tall? Does she walk straight with purpose? Is she strong? Does she have a sense of balance and poise?

Now imagine an unhealthy person as he walks toward you. Is he lethargic as he plods toward you? Are his shoulders slouched and his head down? Does his gait remind you of a duck's waddle, with his feet pointed out and his weight shifting from foot to foot?

I used to do a fat person's duck waddle as my weight prompted me to sway from side to side as I walked. No wonder I was constantly off balance!

Which person are you? Whether you are at the beginning of your journey toward health or far down the road, you can be the athlete.

Your posture doesn't just affect the way you look. It affects the way you feel! If you carry yourself as defeated and fat, you're not likely to want to work out, eat healthy, or consider yourself a success. Likewise, if you carry yourself as healthy, strong, and focused, you'll approach a workout, a meal, and life with confidence.

Throughout the day, do a conscious check to make sure you're walking tall with your head up and focused. Feel the balance and poise that you've developed over these past months. Move with a sense of purpose and reflecting the fact that you are a healthy individual.

Keeping your "eyes fixed on Jesus", how do you hold your head? Your movement reflects your beliefs and your beliefs affect the actions you'll take. Move strong!

Week 12 Day 4: *Journal*

How would you rate your posture today, on a scale of one to ten?

1 _____ 10

What is one simple action that you can do to improve your posture?

_____

_____

_____

Gaining a sense of balance and poise, and carrying yourself with strength is a major benefit of gaining health. Walk with confidence knowing that yours is a life well lived!

✦ Today's Sabai CORE:

C – Cardio Movement   _____

O – Optimum Hydration _____

R – Rest and Recovery _____

E – Eat Healthy   _____

Week 12 Day 5: *Humility*

"God opposes the proud but gives grace to the humble." 1st Peter 5:5b

You've gained health and excess weight has come off. Stay humble.

One morning Cindy and I had planned to run, which I was really excited about because being together with her and challenging each other with our running pace is really fun. Instead, we woke though to the sound of a steady drizzle of rain.

We reconsidered our workout plan. "Let's do Tae Bo", Cindy said. "We haven't done that together in a while!" I have to admit that my response was less than enthusiastic. I'm embarrassed to admit, but I thought I had "graduated" from Tae Bo as I'd lost this weight.

You see, Tae Bo was one of the exercises that I could do when I was severely obese and over 300 lbs. Well, I couldn't do it at the same pace as Billy Blanks, but I could do the routine at a 1/2 speed pace, get a great workout, burn calories, and see improvement over time. Somehow I had decided that my preparation for a triathlon by swimming, biking, and running was much more effective exercise and a better workout. WRONG!

We started the workout. My goodness! Within minutes I was at 120 beats per minutes and then the real workout began. A few minutes later, I glanced at my heart rate monitor and it registered 149 beats per minute! In the months since I did Tae Bo last, I'd forgotten what a fun workout it is. Billy Blanks is always so encouraging and I was amazed that after losing the weight, I can do the workout at full speed, rather than my old 1/2 speed pace.

What an awesome workout and I promise. I will not "dis" Tae Bo again! Stay humble…

Week 12 Day 5: *Journal*

List an exercise that you've "graduated" from over the past three months: *Example: Tae Bo*

Exercise: _____

Choose a day to do that workout and note any changes you'll make, if needed, to intensify the challenge. *Example: Try to keep up with the full pace on the video.*

_____

_____

_____

Movement is movement and exercise is exercise. Enjoy and acknowledge all of your workouts regardless of the challenge level. Balance is created when there is a blending of challenge levels and the net result is fun!

✦ Today's Sabai CORE:

C – Cardio Movement   _____

O – Optimum Hydration   _____

R – Rest and Recovery   _____

E – Eat Healthy   _____

WEEK 12 DAY 6: *Honor the Past*

Joshua told them, "Go in front of the ark of the Lord your God to the middle of the Jordan. Each of you is to put a stone on his shoulder, according to the number of the Israelite tribes. The stones will be a reminder to you. When your children ask someday, 'Why are these stones important to you?' tell them how the water of the Jordan stopped flowing before the ark of the covenant of the Lord. When it crossed the Jordan, the water of the Jordan stopped flowing. These stones will be a lasting memorial for the Israelites." Joshua 4:5-7 (NET)

The healthy response to change is to appreciate the past and the lessons that have been learned. This book came into being because the milestones and lessons learned were recorded along the way!

What a blessing you have by writing this journal over the past 12 weeks! As you've seen your health increase and your weight decrease, what are the lessons you've learned? I have no doubt that each person who arrives at Week 12 Day 7 could write a book of their own!

At the end of the *Biggest Loser* series, contestants are brought face to face with a cardboard cutout of the old body. The reactions are varied from disgust to love to curiosity to disbelief. Love yourself. It is okay to disagree with decisions you made in the past. What's not ok is to minimize or put down your old self. You were doing your best with the knowledge and tools you had. You're different now. You've learned new lessons and come to expect different things from your body. You treat your body with a renewed respect.

Without honoring the past, we are likely to repeat past mistakes. By acknowledging the past and remembering where we came from, we keep ourselves on a great path and focus on where we're going.

Love the person that stood up to the challenge and began this journey. Honor yourself and acknowledge your accomplishments. Loving others will come more naturally when you love yourself.

Acknowledge and honor your past and it will serve you well.

WEEK 12 DAY 6: *Journal*

Write a love note to yourself. What are you most proud of accomplishing in this journey? What changes are you excited to see?

_____

_____

_____

_____

_____

_____

_____

_____

_____

By loving yourself, you'll be honoring the gift of life that God has given you.

✦ Today's Sabai CORE:

C – Cardio Movement   _____

O – Optimum Hydration   _____

R – Rest and Recovery   _____

E – Eat Healthy   _____

WEEK 12 DAY 7: *Pass it on!*

> *"Finally, brothers and sisters, whatever is true, whatever is worthy of respect, whatever is just, whatever is pure, whatever is lovely, whatever is commendable, if something is excellent or praiseworthy, think about these things. And what you learned and received and heard and saw in me, do these things. And the God of peace will be with you." Philippians 4:8-9 (NET)*

Why did you start this journey? Perhaps you wanted to look great for your spouse. Perhaps you wanted to prepare for summer swimsuit season. Perhaps you wanted to be healthy and feel strong again. Whatever the reason, as you've persisted through twelve weeks of lessons and applied them into your own life, you've gained health and insight into your body and mind.

Now, what will you do with it?

My first prayer is that you will continue your journey with open eyes of wonder. Enjoy the new sights and challenges you meet along the way. Revel in the splendor of your body as it was created to be.

My second prayer is that you will share the unique lessons that you've learned. Encourage others who see the path as too difficult. Give someone else the tools that have made a difference to you.

Each day you come in contact with other people who are hurting. Life is filled with gifts and challenges, discouragement and encouragement. Give the gift of encouragement to others. Help make their day a bit brighter and given them hope that they too can find the path.

When you see that person in the gym or the grocery store or at church, notice the weight loss, the healthy glow of their skin, the sparkle in their eye and acknowledge it.

You have been given a precious gift of life and health.

Share it with others and live in love.

WEEK 12 DAY 7: *Journal*

What are some ways that you can help others in this journey? Who is someone you've met over the past twelve weeks that you could encourage? Write down your plan for passing on this gift to others.

_____

_____

_____

When you've gained knowledge, you've also gained a responsibility to share that knowledge. Other people are looking for leadership and encouragement to accomplish their goals. Take another person under your wing and bless them with your time, encouragement, and prayers.

◆ Today's Sabai CORE:

C – Cardio Movement   _____

O – Optimum Hydration   _____

R – Rest and Recovery   _____

E – Eat Healthy   _____

12 Week Measurements: Celebrate!

Date:___/___/___

Twelve weeks ago you started this journey, not quite sure where the road would take you. Celebrate as you take these measurements, remembering that this is not the end of your journey, but only the beginning.

Weight:_____

One mile or kilometer timed:_____

Waist:_____

Chest:_____

How long can you balance on one leg? _____

Look back at your Week 7 Day 2 journal to see your improvement.

Any other measurements you'd like to take:

_____

_____

_____

FINAL THOUGHTS:

You are so amazing! Whether it took you twelve weeks to finish this book or twice as long, it doesn't matter. You've persevered and been faithful to the journey. Along the way, you've learned important lessons and applied them to your life. You've spent time focused on truth, forgiveness, discipline, and honor.

Acknowledge the strides that you've made. Look forward with anticipation to the changes that await you as you continue on your journey.

While you are at the end of this book, you are also at beginning of your journey. Together we have walked the first miles and charted new territory. What's really important is the book that you write with the lessons that you learn. Make note of the lessons that you learn along the way. What are the truths that you discover that you want to share with the world?

I'd invite you to send the lessons you learn to me at: lessons@healthasmission.com Perhaps one day your lesson will be part of a follow up book in this series!

Use your knowledge to bless others. As you build into yourself, use the energy gained to help those around you. Working together, we can accomplish great things. Choose to make a difference in the lives of others.

APPENDIX A: SALVATION PLAN

STEPS TO PEACE WITH GOD

1. RECOGNIZE GOD'S PLAN—PEACE AND LIFE

   The message in this book stresses that God loves you
   and wants you to experience His peace and life.

   The BIBLE says ... For God loved the
   world so much that He gave His only Son,
   so that everyone who believes in Him may
   not die but have eternal life. John 3:16

2. REALIZE OUR PROBLEM—SEPARATION

   People choose to disobey God and go their
   own way. This results in separation from God.

   The BIBLE says ... Everyone has
   sinned and is far away from God's saving
   presence. Romans 3:23

3. RESPOND TO GOD'S REMEDY—CROSS OF CHRIST

   God sent His Son to bridge the gap. Christ
   did this by paying the penalty of our sins when
   He died on the cross and rose from the grave.

   The BIBLE says ... But God has shown
   us how much He loves us—it was while we
   were still sinners that Christ died for us!
   Romans 5:8

   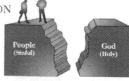

4. RECEIVE GOD'S SON—LORD AND SAVIOR

   You cross the bridge into God's family when
   you ask Christ to come into your life.

   The BIBLE says ... Some, however, did
   receive Him and believed in Him; so He
   gave them the right to become God's
   children. John 1:12

   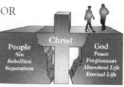

THE INVITATION IS TO:

REPENT (turn from your sins) and by faith RECEIVE Jesus Christ into your heart
and life and follow Him in obedience as your Lord and Savior.

PRAYER OF COMMITMENT

"Dear Lord Jesus, I know that I am a sinner, and I ask for Your forgiveness. I believe
You died for my sins and rose from the dead. I turn from my sins and invite You to
come into my heart and life. I want to trust and follow You as my Lord and Savior.
In Your Name, Amen."

If you are committing your life to Christ, please let us know!

Billy Graham Evangelistic Association
1 Billy Graham Parkway, Charlotte, NC 28201-0001
1-877-2GRAHAM (1-877-247-2426)
billygraham.org

APPENDIX B: CONTACT INFORMATION

WILLIAM HAYNES

301 Poinsettia Drive
Simpsonville, SC 29681
william@sabaifitness.com
www.sabaifitness.com

Notes:

Notes:

Notes:

Notes: